Shout Outs

I want to give thanks and praise to the most high God for allowing me put these thoughts on paper and share them with His creations. I pray that He is pleased with this book and allows people to use this as an aid to help them honor their body as a temple of His Spirit.

I also want to give thanks to my lovely and awesome wife who makes it possible for me to kick butt in life, my Pastor for all his help in life, his Pastor for the same, Momma I for pushing me hard to always do my best, Momma G for helping me get closer to God, and all of my family who God uses to make me a stronger man.

Edited By: Bishop Terry Gilmore, Barbara Iacino, Barbara Johannessen Bailey, and Maile Stricker

Table of Contents

Our company started offering weight loss coaching for employee health programs and we needed a diet that worked. At the same time I was motivated to lose weight, so out of those two motives "The Fist Diet" was born.

The Fist Diet is a program that focuses on human nature rather than on robotic regimens. It is designed not as a weight loss technique but as a way of life. Since eating is a part of our everyday life and always will be, it was important to develop a system that was achievable throughout one's entire lifespan. The Fist Diet is doable, sustainable, and non-burdensome. It was created to lose weight and maintain that healthy weight for the rest of one's life.

The key to the Fist Diet's success is that it does not demonize or restrict certain foods, thus giving the user the power to eat whatever they want.

When we first developed the Fist Diet I volunteered to be the first guinea pig. I weighed 220 lbs. at the time. When I got married in my early 20s I weighed 165 lbs. The added weight was not from body building either. I gained 10 lbs when I got married. Another 10 lbs. when I got promoted to a charge nurse and had to work the night shift. I gained 10 lbs. with the birth of each one of my 3 kids and the last ten was from stress and trash food eating.

I wanted to get back into fighting shape. I was on prescription proton pump inhibitors for severe chronic heart burn, I got beaten in a race by a 15 year old, I lost my swagger and mojo when I was decked out in my church suits, and I was used to being the "go to guy" for health information and now people were taking advice from others who were giving them less than sound advice. It was all building up and let's just say I was motivated for change.

I started on the Fist Diet in January 2012. I started losing up to 5 lbs. a week. In six months I was down 60 lbs. to a weight of 160 lbs.

I will share this logical, factual, scientific weight loss strategy that is embedded with psychology with all of you.

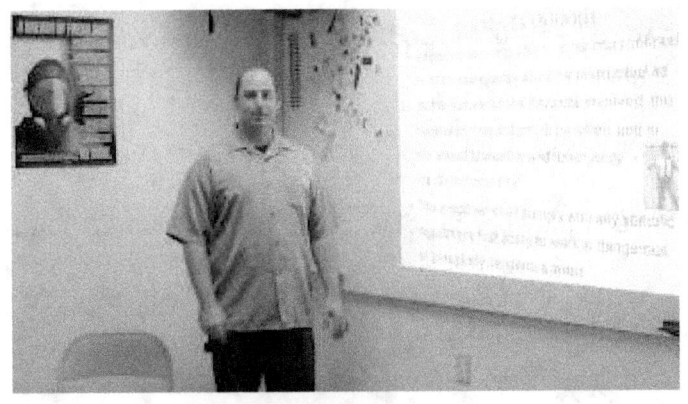

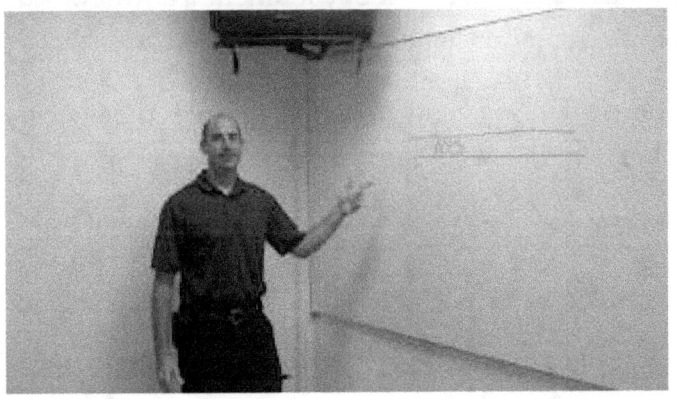

Do you feel it is extremely difficult to lose weight?

Have you tried countless diets over the years with little or no results?

Have you or are you ready to give up on dieting altogether?

Do you want to take your life back from the burden of complex diet rules?

Do you have an 8 page list of foods that you <u>cannot</u> eat?

Do you have a handful of foods that you <u>are</u> allowed to eat on your current diet?

Do you have to travel with special equipment for your diet?

Do you have to lug special "diet" foods with you when you travel?

Are your friends and family tired of having to deal with your stress from trying burdensome diets?

Are you tired of spending most of your mental power on your diet rules, counting and calculating?

Are you tired of feeling guilty for failing at a diet that is impossible or improbable to follow to begin with?

Are you ready to succeed?

Are you ready to keep it off?

Are you ready to start enjoying life?

Are you ready to take your life back?

Are you ready to search for motivation?

Are you ready to make a decision?

Then start saving money for a new wardrobe and to get your rings resized. The Fist Diet is here and can help you achieve your goals.

To start the Fist Diet you must take the following steps of mental preparation:

1. Find a reason to stop overeating

2. Find a motivation to not eat worthless foods
3. Learn/understand what it means to overeat
4. Learn/understand what a worthless food is
5. Learn/understand what a calorie containing food is
6. Learn/understand what a negative and zero calorie containing food is
7. Learn the nutrition basics of vitamins, minerals, fats, carbs, and proteins

Once you have mastered these Fist Diet fundamentals, you can begin your journey to the new you. You will be like a new person because you may have felt and looked this good before but never with the knowledge and experience you now have. Sure, you can get down to the weight you were in your early 20s but now you will have the know-how to accomplish previously unimaginable things.

FAD = Failure Already Determined

Choosing a diet should be like choosing your mate. Ask yourself, am I prepared to live with this person/diet for the rest of my life? Ask yourself if you can sustain this new Hollywood trendy diet forever? Because once you quit the fad diet the weight will come back as fast as it went or faster, this is called recidivism.

So diets that make you give up food or eat and drink really weird things will usually only last a month or so.

Definition of Diet

•A: Food and drink regularly provided or consumed

•B: Habitual nourishment

•C: The kind and amount of food prescribed for a person or animal for a special reason

D: A regimen of eating and drinking sparingly so as to reduce one's weight <going on a diet>

•E: Something provided or experienced repeatedly <a diet of Broadway shows and nightclubs — Frederick Wyatt>

Source - Webster's Dictionary

Every human is on a diet. Our diet is what we eat normally/consistently. So when we try a fad "diet" for a month or so, it really is not our diet. Our diet is what we return to eating when we quit our fad "diet". Our routine consistent diet is what makes us over, under, or a healthy weight.

So what is your diet? What do you eat consistently? How is it treating you? Are you at your ideal body image?

Origin of the word DIET:
It comes from the Middle English word diete, from Anglo-French, from Latin diaeta, from Greek diaita, literally, means the manner of living, from diaitasthai to lead one's life

First Known Use: 13th century
Source - Webster's Dictionary

Definition of Food

A: Material consisting essentially of protein, carbohydrate, and fat used in the body of an organism to sustain growth, repair, and vital processes and to furnish energy; also: such food together with supplementary substances (as minerals, vitamins, and condiments)

B: Inorganic substances absorbed by plants in gaseous form or in water solution

C: Nutriment in solid form

D: Something that nourishes, sustains, or supplies <food for thought>

Source - Webster's Dictionary

Notice that food is not defined as entertainment, celebration tool, or anxiety and depression remedy. Food is fuel. Food is the gasoline for our motor. Just because you get your actual gas from a gas station, does not mean that you have to get your meals there too.

Are you fit? Here is an enlightening definition I pulled out of my old nutrition book from the nursing program.

Fitness Defined

1. Flexible Joints
2. Muscle strength and endurance
3. Heart strength and endurance
4. Healthy body composition
5. Able to perform daily activities with enough energy to handle an emergency

6. Able to withstand physiological and psychological stresses
Source: Understanding Nutrition Seventh Edition

Overetiology: 1. The reasons we overeat; 2. the way we overeat

Negative calories

Negative calorie foods rock! They are a total life saver for all those who eat fruit and vegetables and who are trying to lose weight. A negative calorie food is one that takes your body more or equal calories to digest it than that are contained in them.

So if the fruit or vegetable has 50 calories in it and it takes our body 55 calories to digest or metabolize it, then the snack is actually negative calories.

How can this be, you ask? Plant matter has a matrix. Plants get their shape from strands called cellulose. We humans get our matrix or shape from our bones, tendons, ligaments, and muscles. Cellulose is like plant bones. When we eat the whole fruit or vegetable we ingest their matrix too. You have all seen the stuff; the strings on the banana when you peel it, the plasticy stuff around each wedge of an orange slice, the stringy stuff in celery that gets caught in your teeth. It's all plant bones. These plant bones are hard to digest and some are indigestible and otherwise known as dietary fiber. So when you eat them it takes longer for your body to break them down. The effort your digestive system is exerting requires calories to fuel the process, thus you are burning calories just after you ingested calories.

The calories you burn from the digestion of this plant matter are not the same calories from the plant you ingested but rather sugar that was already in your blood stream. The natural fructose you ingested from your apple is cancelled out by the glucose in your blood that was used as fuel to break down the apples bones.

Drinking fruit juice is the fastest way to get sugar into your blood stream without a needle involved. Fruit juice is loaded with carbs and will definitely affect your waistline if you are consuming large quantities daily. So why is apple juice bad for the waistline and a whole apple is not? The answer is twofold: First, you are not getting any of the plant bones in the juice; it has been all processed out. So, you do not have to use any calories to break it down. There is virtually nothing to break down. Second, the manufacturers probably added some sugar for taste.

Phases of the Fist Diet

There are three phases of the Fist Diet. Here is a synopsis of all three. Phase 1: Eat less. Phase 2: Eat less and eat better. Phase 3: Eat less, eat better and exercise.

Fence Riding Explained

"Fence Riding" is when a person who has been on multiple diets does not stick to one plan. They take several different components of past diets and put them all together. This usually leads to weight gain.

For example if you were on a low to no carb diet for a long time, it was OK in that diet's regimen to eat hot dogs because they have low or no carbs. So for months to years you programmed your brain that hot dogs were "good" or "healthy". Now that you are on the Fist Diet, it is still programmed in your mind that hot dogs are "good". When you have consumed your three fist sized portions of calorie containing foods for the day and you are still hungry you turn to your good old buddy the hot dog because it is on your "OK to eat" list.

To fully get the benefit of any diet plan you have to work the diet's rules. For example if you are on a low to no carb diet, then you cannot eat carbs. If you break the diet's rules you will not be able to tap into the weight loss benefits of the diet's design.

So what do you do? Find a diet that is both healthy and realistic and stick to it. Too often people break the diet's rules and then blame the diet for not working.

This is one of the beauties of the Fist Diet. The rules are simple and it is very doable to anyone with the motivation. You don't have a ten page list of foods you can never eat again. Meat is not the enemy. Carbs are not the enemy. Food is not the enemy. How we misuse and overeat food is the enemy.

Do you find yourself doing this? Ask yourself "how is it working"? "Are you losing weight"?

Worthless/Trash Food Explained (A.K.A. Junk Food)

A worthless/trash food is: 1) A substance that only benefits the taste buds but has no positive health benefits (soda)

2) A substance that has little to no nutritional value and has negative health consequences (alcohol, energy drinks.)

3) Has an extremely high glycemic index meaning it immediately turns into sugar, spiking one's blood sugar, which causes a secretion of insulin, which causes a hypoglycemic crash after the insulin pulls all the sugar into the cells, and causes a rapid hunger return to get more sugar back into the blood stream.

Examples: chips, doughnuts, candy, white rice, white bread, most fast food...

Balance

- To gain weight: eat more calories than you will burn
- To maintain weight: eat the same amount of calories as you burn
- To lose weight: eat fewer calories than you burn

It's like a house full of clutter; we are overweight because we get new stuff faster than we have garage sales. We ingest more calories than we burn and all the extra calories are converted to fat.

Psychology and Logic

What is the purpose of food?

- Nourishment
- Sustain life
- Fuel

What do we use food for? Why are we eating what we are eating? Why are we eating when we are eating? I'm guessing and going off my personal experience, that 75% of the time we are doing these things for the wrong reason.

If we are truly eating to sustain our lives and for nourishment then we wouldn't be eating this over processed garbage that we do. So there must be a psychological reason for our eating habits. For me it was stress eating and boredom eating. I also overate a lot of junk to compromise with my flesh. I deny my flesh on so many things that I guess I didn't want to fight it when it came time to eat too. So I gave in and gave it whatever it wanted and as much as it wanted. Before I knew it I was a big ball of flesh. I fed my flesh and flesh grew.

Overeating

We are all overeaters. We think of overeaters as 400-500 pound people with zero self-control; however the average American overeats at every meal. We easily consume over 670 calories per meal. Some of us eat more than that not only for three meals a day but for four meals a day. A 12 once pop can has turned into a liter bottle. A large pop at the drive through is now the same size as a mega gulp. If we go out to eat we could consume 2000 calories in one setting. We should be eating enough food at a mealtime to carry us to our next meal; however we normally eat enough food to carry us into next week.

Overeating is simply consuming more calories than your body requires to run. This is why America is overweight; we eat high calorie, fast burning, worthless foods in large amounts.

We may only eat 2000 calories a day, but some of us drink 2000 calories a day as well.

"You are what you ate", not "You are what you eat". What we eat today is not the reason we are overweight. We are overweight because of what we have eaten every day for the past several years.

We overeat because: Pleasure, anti-depressant, anti-anxiety medicine, stress medicine, coping skill, boredom cure, entertainment, medicine side effects, learned behavior, culture, availability, peer pressure, self-medication, no hope of getting in shape due to disability, grief, celebration, or out of habit.

We abuse and misuse food. Our appetite is a learned response to our life up to this point. Take a minute to think who you learned it from and how they are faring health wise.

Motivated vs. Disciplined

We will cover many different motivating factors to eat less and to eat better: On the market, Pride, Health, Money, Time, Fun, Control, and Sex Life.

Hopefully you will find a motivating factor that hits home to you? If not it is OK as long as you find the one that you want more than you want to overeat and eat worthless foods.

Without the proper motivation no diet will work for you. I don't care if it is the "eat cake diet"; you will break it after two days to eat an apple if you are not motivated to lose weight.

People have told me that I must have a great deal of discipline to follow a diet for this long and to lose the amount of weight that I did. People have told me that they could never do what I did because they do not have the discipline.

My response to them is that for the Fist Diet there is no discipline required, just a strong motivation.

Every time we are faced with an opportunity to overeat we just have to remember our motivating factors. Every time we want to eat worthless foods we have to remember why we want to lose weight. If that motivating factor is more desirable to us than that doughnut or bag of chips, then we will walk by it.

If we do not find the motivation, we will never lose the weight unless we go through a terrible depressive phase or get really sick.

Motivation

All you need to do to transform your body is to find a strong enough motivation. The Fist Diet is a rapid weight loss plan for those who have found a strong motivation.

Weak or no motivation = no change in body

What is your motivation?

On the market (Single)

Pride

Health/Fear

Money

Time

Fun

Control

Sex Life

People think dieting is all about discipline. Are you disciplined enough not to walk down a dark alley at night? No you are motivated to live and do not want to die in a mugging gone wrong. Will you be disciplined enough to turn down those doughnuts and chips? Ask anyone who has went from an unhealthy weight to a healthy weight and kept it off. They will all tell you that they stay on the path for a specific reason, a specific motivating factor. They will each probably give you a different reason or motivating factor. Your motivating factor might be different from theirs. The point is to dig deep a find a powerful enough reason to quit overeating. We as humans get everything we want. We just have to want to be at a healthy weight more than we want the temporary pleasure of overeating. To accomplish this we have to find the reasons we need to be at a healthy weight. That is our motivation.

Market Motivation

Are you looking for your other half?

Getting healthy and to your ideal shape will boost your self-esteem and confidence. These two factors will help you say what you need to say to communicate your affection.

Realizing your ideal body image is one of the greatest ways to boost your self-esteem. Low self-esteem is one of the biggest obstacles in making a move on the person of your interest. Low self-esteem =

lower chance of asking them out. You will never make them your other half without going for it.

When the weight loss ball starts rolling it rolls into other aspects of our lives as well, I noticed when I started losing weight that I starting taking better care of my teeth, dressing better, and making sure my hair was cut on time. Before, I wasn't as motivated to keep myself up, but once you start taking care of yourself in one aspect the rest of the body wants to jump on the let's get "GQ" train.

Pride Motivation

Are you unable to do the physical things that you used to do due to your weight?

This was me all to pieces. I couldn't stretch the way I used to with this new gut in the way. I couldn't last as long while playing with my kids, and I lost a race to a 15 year old. All the extra weight I had picked up was causing joint pain which made me want to be active less.

So it was a downward spiral. The more I weighed, the less I wanted to be active. The less I was active, the more I would weigh.

These issues were some of my biggest motivators to stop overeating and to stop eating trash food. I decided that I wanted to be physically active more than I wanted to continue my unhealthy eating habits.

Health/Fear Motivation

Why would someone in their right mind ever pass up on fresh made doughnuts or any other of their favorite pastries? Why would you ever put the fork down and push away your plate when it is still full of some awesome and killer food?

These are the answers we must find if we are ever going to lose any weight and keep it off. For me health was one of my biggest motivating factors. I was on a prescription strength proton pump inhibiter for chronic heart burn. All the excess fat I accumulated would crowd my abdominal cavity and push on my stomach. This would cause gastric acid to be forced up my throat (If this goes unchecked it can lead to esophageal cancer). My Doctor and I also discussed some recent studies that have linked these meds to spinal fractures. The theory is that since these meds decrease the amount of stomach acid you produce they decrease digestion of calcium. With less and less calcium in your system the taker becomes more susceptible to spinal fractures.

Needless to say this was not on my agenda. I knew that when I weighed less than 200lbs I didn't have the heartburn. So for me losing the weight was a must.

Type 2 Diabetes in America is at an all-time high with more and more kids and adults being diagnosed every day. The crazy thing is they are in a similar boat as I was. If they lose the excess weight their Diabetes will go away!

Fear is one of the most powerful forces of motivation on the planet, whether human or animal. When the Doctor tells you that "you are going to die a lot sooner if you don't lose weight", it will motivate some to change their lifestyle. I have seen people who smoked cigarettes for 40 years quit after having a heart attack. Before the heart attack, they tried hundreds of times to quit smoking. So, what worked this time? The answer is fear. Fear of death to be more specific. I have also seen people quit their fast food chains after almost dying from clogged arteries. Why this time? Fear of death.

Are you afraid of dying due to all the health complications caused from excess body fat? If you have enough fear, you will have the motivation to change your lifestyle and start losing weight.

Here are some other reasons or motivating factors to stop overeating and eating worthless nutrient free foods.

- Lower cholesterol
- Lower blood pressure
- Get off the medications
- Lower cancer risks: colon, esophageal, etc...
- Lower heart attack risk
- Lower common colds by increasing immunity
- Eradicate disease causing fat
- Get rid of Type 2 Diabetes altogether
- Increase weight = increased death rate

Financial Motivation

I know people who will only move when they can see a financial reason to. Here some financial reasons to stop overeating and eating worthless foods. By the way, overeating not only costs more at the store but it cost us thousands in copays and in medical bills. So if you are looking for a monetary return on investment to stop eating too much think about the loads of dough you'll save on health care. I personally save about $50.00 a week from not eating out as much. I also save $10.00 on month from one prescription I don't need anymore. Here are some money motivators for you:

- Eating out once will now last for three meals
- Grocery money will stretch
- More time on the clock
- Less or zero medications
- Make more money at work due to your ability to do more work physically and mentally
- Increase of fat can = increase of insurance premiums
- Increase in fat can be a factor in job and social discrimination

Time Motivation

When you eat appropriate sized portions you will find more time in your day due to:

- Less time eating
- Less time in the bathroom
- Less time making food
- Less time waiting for food at restaurants
- Less time at the Doctor due to your health problems caused by excess fat
- Less time taking medications for problems caused by excess body weight
- Less time performing physical chores
- Less recovery time after performing physical chores
- Less time trying to find money for bills because you saved lots of money not eating out as much

Fun Motivation

My fun time with my kids lasts so much longer now and is such a better quality. I can actually tire them out now. Before, I would have to take several rest breaks during play time. Sometimes I couldn't even start the play time because I was in joint pain.

When we were young we thought our dad was superman because of the things he could physically do. I am superman again in my kid's eyes.

Do you want to be able to play with your children or grandchildren for longer periods of time?

Do you want to be able to partake in the physical activities of your interest?

I have been able to partake in activities I enjoyed in my youth. Climbing rock walls, running a mile, mountain biking etc... I had previously given up on most physical hobbies due to my overweight condition.

Control Motivation

Kids may not have control over when they eat or what is served at school or at home. As adults we also may have limited control over the food we eat due to poor accessibility of nutrient dense foods and limited financial resources.

We may not have control over what we eat, when we eat, financial resources for the food we buy to eat, but we do have control over how much we eat.

So if all we have to eat is greasy fried foods, we can at least make sure we are not overeating those foods. We can still lose weight eating those kinds of foods as long as we are not consuming too much of them. Of course malnourishment is always a concern so it is important that we make every effort possible to speak up that we want real food.

Sex Life

You guessed it. Even our most intimate moments are negatively affected by our overeating. I like eating probably more than the next guy, however I like this topic more than eating the best foods on the planet. So why do we chose the pleasure of overeating over great cleaving time with our spouse? Is it because we fail to make the connection between our overeating and what goes on or doesn't go on in the bedroom?

Impotence is prevalent with overweight males. The cause of impotence can be traced back to many different roots, both psychological and physiological. Let's deal with psychological first.

Confidence:

When we are overweight it is hard for us to believe that our mate wants to sleep with us. When we don't feel sexy we won't initiate or reciprocate our spouse's advances. The extra weight can make the physical act difficult leading to less and less confidence. If we want to continue to make love to our spouse, then we have to choose them over the spoon.

Now let's cover some of the physiological reasons for impotence.

Polycythemia is thick blood. Polycythemia can be caused from having too much body fat or too much sugar floating around in your vessels due to diabetes.

For every pound of fat we gain our bodies must supply that new tissue with blood to keep it alive. So our body has to produce more blood vessels and the heart has to work even harder to pump blood to and through the new fat.

Thick blood as well as the heart's heavy work load of getting blood through all the fat tissues makes it hard to form an erection.

No Patience Required

It took you years to gain the weight and it's going to take time to lose it. However if you find a powerful motivation, by following the Fist Diet you will lose approximately 10-20 pounds a month.

Patience is an area I am always working on. When I got motivated to lose weight I didn't want a diet that was going to take me one to two years to get me where I wanted to be. I knew that I had gained 60 pounds in 10 years but I definitely didn't want to take ten years to lose it.

When I started the Fist Diet, I started to see immediate results. I was losing three to five pounds a week. After six months I had lost the weight I had gained in ten years.

Immediate results are very important to keep us those of us who are challenged in the patience department from getting discouraged. Many people quit working diets because they get discouraged about slow results. We are a "got to have it now" generation and with the Fist Diet you can lose weight healthy and fast.

Fist Psych

As you start the Fist Diet and force your body to burn the excess fat, your body will resist.

Your mind will play tricks on you. Your body will act as though it is dying. Your body will send you a sensation that you have never felt before to try to trick you that it is serious enough for you to start over eating. This is a mind battle. Our flesh (AKA human nature) is the enemy.

We need to take this one meal at a time. Every meal time is game time. We have to remember our motivations and not overeat.

Snack time is battle time. We have to battle our old unhealthy habits and chose negative or zero calorie snacks.

Not only are our eyes bigger than our stomachs, so are our emotions. When we eat according to our emotional state we will always overeat and usually eat trash foods.

It takes time for food to move through our gastrointestinal tract .

Eat slowly; If we slow down and eat slowly, not only will we actually taste our food, we will give ample time for our stomachs to send signals to our brains of food arriving.

Give meal time the respect it deserves. If we eat in the car, while we are on the computer, while we are watching TV, we will not focus on the food. That means we won't be conscious of how much we are eating and we won't enjoy it either. If we don't have a mental grasp on what we ate, we are more prone to eat more at the next meal to compensate.

Feeling full can be just as much mental as physical. Let us focus on the food at meal time. Then we will know that we have consumed enough when that hunger feeling comes around later. We can use that logic to tell our stomach to shut up because we know that we have consumed adequate amounts to sustain us until the next meal.

We have accepted and become OK with being overweight. Complacency is one of the biggest obstacles in overcoming change. If you don't want to change you never will. If you are OK with all of problems your overeating has caused you then there is nothing I could say to motivate you. Some of us however are just so discouraged with dieting that we stopped believing we can lose weight altogether. Some of us have been overweight for so long that we forgot how miserable it makes us.

We have accepted our shape as "cursed genes". 95% of us do not have genetic obesity. Please let us all stop blaming our genes. True, you have a genetic predisposition to carry excess weight in certain places on your body, so all the overweight people in your family will have the same shape. That is not cursed genes. The genes told your body where to store the excess fat, they didn't make the fat, we did.

Sometimes we chose to stay overweight because it is a "get out of jail free card". I see this in kids most often but I have seen plenty of adults use their weight and health to get out of everything from manual labor to taking certain titles. Kids will use their weight to get out of physical education type of events, which of course helps keep them overweight.

Being overweight can keep the opposite sex away. In my decade of Psyc Nursing I have worked with a lot of females who have been sexually assaulted. Some of them purposefully become and stay overweight and also try to keep their appearances less than attractive to ward off potential perpetrators. To them I say spend the same amount of time learning Muay Thai kickboxing, Jujitsu grappling, Mace techniques, take and master the skills taught in a "Refuse To Be A Victim" class, rather than hurting yourself as a defensive mechanism. Point being that there are healthier and more effective ways to make sure that those horrible things never happen to you again.

Sometimes we stay overweight because it gets us attention. Even a mom, sister, aunt, or doctor nagging at us due to our weight could actually be welcomed attention to the right person. I say get attention in a healthier way. Drop the pounds and do something incredible with your new found energy and the attention will come. At the very least you will get more attention from the weight loss than you ever did from overeating.

Starting Fist Psych

Don't "player hate" the over eaters: Once you stop overeating, it will become painfully obvious when someone else is overeating. It's like when you quit smoking, you didn't mind the smell before but now it is repulsive. You also noticed everybody that is smoking where you didn't before. Try your best not to get on the people around you for overeating and for consuming way more calories than they will burn that day. Instead let your looks do the convicting/convincing. Once you start shedding the weight they will slowly start to see how much they are consuming.

Don't brag. This is extremely hard. After the first ten comes off, then twenty, then thirty, you will want to tell the whole world. You will want everyone else to lose weight because you found a way that was so easy and really works. You will want everyone to feel the way you do. If we do this overzealously we will be in the same classification as dental hygienists and lactation specialists. It's not a religion and people can stay over weight if they want to. It will be hard to not preach at your loved one who has been trying to lose weight forever. It will be difficult to hear the complaints about weight related medical issues from the people in your life when you found a way out for them and they refuse to get on the same path. But moral of the story is to focus on you. Be an example. Hopefully you will inspire them. But it can back fire on us if we beat them over the head with it.

Remember your motivation every time you are tempted to overeat. When you first get started it will be hard to break old habits. It gets easier as you go. The less you weigh the less your body needs to survive. The less you will be hungry. Once you start you will need to really focus otherwise you will forget and overeat. So, every meal remember your motivation to lose weight and push the plate away after you have consumed a fist size of calorie containing foods.

When I first started on the Fist Diet I needed a crutch. I didn't have a good grasp on zero and negative calorie options. I did know that most pickles were zero calorie, so I would eat a ton of pickles with my meals to still feel like I was getting enough content. This was OK for me until I learned about my other options, but if you need to watch your salt intake I would go with veggies that weren't soaked in salty brine.

Write your motivating factors down and place them where you will see them every day, both at home and at work. It is a good idea to have a constant reminder why you are turning down all this temporary pleasure of overeating. After a few weeks however, you will be too busy having fun on the scale to ever want to overeat again.

Expect to be "player hated" and not complimented. This, ladies and gentleman, is the reason behind the name of the book **Fitness Prejudice The Fist Diet**. When I started losing weight people did nothing but insult and "player hate" me. I took flak from every direction. Close friends, family, work, everywhere. They did nothing but make fun of me and try to make me cave and return to the buffet. I had an easier time being a vegetarian in the Midwest than I had losing weight.

Back home we call this the ghetto mentality. It is where no one wants you to succeed in life because you will leave the projects and leave them and will take away their excuses. Elsewhere they call it the cockroach syndrome. If you put a bunch of roaches in an opened top jar, they will all want out but won't work together to get out. Instead they will trample and hinder each other. So our motivation factor has to be stronger than our insecurities, because **you will** be "player hated" and if you want to reach your weight or ideal body shape goal then you will have to endure the insults.

More Fist Psych

We learned earlier what the definition of food is. So it shouldn't be a surprise to learn that food is not for satisfaction. Good food however, is incredibly satisfying. There is nothing wrong with enjoying food, actually, if you are into good tasting quality foods (a foodie), then losing weight can be easier for you. It will be easier to turn down low quality foods. It's as if you are saving the calories you are going to ingest for some worthy food. It's OK to be a food snob. Don't eat everything that is made available to you. Just because there is free food at work today, does not mean you have to eat it. Just because a co-worker brought in a box of gas station doughnuts does not mean that you have to eat them.

Even though good quality food is satisfying, it should not be in the top five satisfiers of our life. We should get our satisfaction from life itself: service, accomplishments, family, careers, transforming our bodies and minds, hobbies, etc...

The Disservice of Eating To Be Full

We do not need to eat to feel full. If we eat until we feel full, we have over-eaten. Being full is more mental than physical. We need to eat portions based on facts instead of feelings. Feelings are tied to emotions; we can't use our emotions as an intake gauge. Our stomachs are only as big as our fists put together. When we overeat, we ingest more than the normal size of our stomach. This causes a signal to be sent to our brain saying STOP. That is how we feel full. There can be a 20 minute lag in that satiety signal. When we are "full" it means that we have over-eaten and stretched our stomach outside of its normal parameters (the size of your two fists put together).

One theory is that the stomach has muscle memory, when we stretch it out, it then expects to get that expanded the next meal. So it will take more and more to feel "full" every time, just like a drug tolerance. So if we are eating until we get that full feeling, then we are overeating more and more and gaining more and more each meal. If we stop eating when we have eaten the right portion size, then we will always know that we did not eat too much.

Reality Escape

Food is not an escape from reality. I know when I would have a large cheese pizza from a killer local pizza joint in front of me, that I was not thinking about my problems. When I was driving while eating two or three double cheeseburgers I was not thinking about bills. But as soon as the eating was over I still had the same problems and now I also feel terrible because I just consumed more than I know I should have.

If our life sucks we need to pinpoint why it sucks and work towards fixing it. The best way to get rid of stress is to attack the root of the stress. The best way to reduce the feeling that our life sucks is to knock out the causes one by one. Sure, eating will give you a brief escape from reality but it will make you worse off than when you started. Think of how we are programmed from society to eat trash when we feel bad. We have been taught to do this from birth. How many movies, TV shows, and comic strips have you seen the female character go binge on a tub of ice cream when she gets dumped? Have you ever done this? Where did you learn to do this? Do we have to respond this way? How about we take all that sadness and frustration out on the pavement or treadmill? This way we can channel that negativity into something positive. We will also look better and feel better. It doesn't hurt either that the "duffus" who dumped you may regret it after he or she sees your rocking new look.

However, if our life is going to take several years to get to a point of some comfort then we need to find healthy escapes; Vacations, hobbies etc... Food is a bad coping skill. There are too many negative consequences that stem from eating to escape.

Food is not entertainment

You do not have to eat while your watch TV or when you are on the computer. If you eat while your brain is preoccupied you will not be able to control your portions well. If you eat while you are on the computer or watching TV, you will overeat. You will consume a whole bag of chips in a one hour show. Plus you will not have fully enjoyed it because you were not focusing on it. That's a double negative, if you are going to hurt yourself eating trash carbs, then you might as well get some pleasure from it.

You should not eat to cure boredom. There are so many healthy things to do when you are bored. Eating to pass time will have too many negative consequences. We should exercise or do something else productive if we are bored.

Food should not be used as an anti-depressant medication

Overeating has and will lead to increased guilt, depression, low self-esteem, decreased energy, decreased motivation, poor self-perception and confidence, physical pain, disease, poor sex life and dissatisfaction with life.

So if we eat to help us become less depressed it will only cause more depression. Most of us do not suffer from a DSM-5 text book diagnosable depression. The average American gets depressed over negative circumstances. If we focus on eradicating those negative circumstances, we will lift the depression. If you do suffer from a clinical depression or a normal depressive moment, getting to your ideal body shape will undoubtedly make you feel better. When we like us, we feel like conquering the world. When we do not like ourselves then we feel like hiding from the world. Getting to a healthy weight will not solve all your problems but it will help you to overcome them.

Food is not a god

We treat food like a god when we turn to it for help, healing, an emotional lift, or joy. Food is a false god that will give you temporary pleasure but multiple long lasting negative consequences. It can be like adultery, temporary pleasure but a life-time of hurt.

So let us turn to the real God for spiritual help and let us refrain from committing food adultery. Meaning that, we avoid the temporary pleasure of over-eating and stick to the plan that will lead to long-lasting happiness. The kind of happiness caused from being healthy and having the energy to live our lives to the fullest.

When we are overweight, we have little to zero energy. We tire too fast and have poor stamina to accomplish much. If we do push ourselves to get a big job done, then we suffer the consequences for a least a week. When we get to a healthy weight not only can we accomplish more but we won't have to pay for it later.

Food is not a reward

We are programmed to use food to celebrate. Every holiday, any time someone graduates, gets married, dies, turns a year older, gets a promotion, closes a deal, buys a house, etc... What do we all do? We go waste a bunch of money hurting ourselves; we all go and "pig out".

We use these moments as excuses to eat in a way we know is unhealthy. These events are terrible on anyone trying to cut the excess fat out of their lives. Sometimes, we can go from one of these events to another and gorge out four times a week. Just because your cousin's kid graduated from high school does not mean you have to overeat. At most of these events there is always an untouched vegetable platter somewhere. Pig out on that. Skip the ranch dressing and go nuts, or at least get some veggies on a plate so you can *"social-eat-alize"* with your family. Eating the veggies will not mess with your diet/lifestyle because they will be zero or negative calorie. Or if you are going to use this food as a meal, grab a fist sized portion of something nutrient dense. Something like chicken breast or a least a three sections of those wrap slices.

Save all the money you would have spent on celebration food and buy yourself something that won't cause guilt, depression, low self-esteem, decreased energy, decreased motivation, poor self-perception and confidence, poor sex life, physical pain, disease and a dissatisfaction with life.

When you want to eat a worthless food ask yourself, would I rather look/feel the way you want to or allow temporary food pleasure to control me?

Celebrate without over-eating. Take the money you spend on restaurants for celebrating and invest in yourself, or save it for a vacation.

Food is not an anti-stress medication

Attack the thing that is causing the stress by planning and hard work. If you cannot eliminate the cause of the stress, then channel that frustration into your workout or another positive coping skill.

Proportionate Portions

Our fist is proportionate to our body size. If you are small framed you will have a small fist. If you are large framed you will have a larger fist. Eating calorie containing foods the size of your fist will be approximately half of your stomach's capacity.

This is the simple beauty of the Fist Diet. No calorie or carb counting. The only calculating you have to do is count to three. Eat portions the size of your fist of calorie containing foods three times a day.

If we were to have a slogan for phase 1 of the Fist Diet, it would be; "Eat Less". You will lose weight if you only eat half of your stomach's capacity three times a day. You will be taking in fewer calories than your body needs to run so your body will have to burn fat to run normally.

This is only dangerous if you have no fat to burn. If you are like the average American, then you have 25-100 excess pounds of fat to burn.

I can't stress enough that the fist size portions are only for calorie containing foods. You can eat a mountain of zero or negative calories foods all day long if you want to. I do recommend eating lots of zero and negative calorie foods both as snacks and with your three meals. This will help four ways: 1. Ensure you are getting enough fiber, 2. Ensure you are getting enough vitamins and minerals, 3. Ensure that you are eating enough content for regularity, and 4. Psychologically it will produce the satiety (full) signal we are used to feeling when we eat.

Phase 1 (Weight Loss)

Eat Less

Imagine if you knew someone that ate five doughnuts for every meal every day. This person would undoubtedly be overweight. Now, let's say this person cut down to one doughnut for every meal three times a day. Wha la, magic this person is dropping weight like crazy. Now he is starting his own diet called the "Doughnut Diet". He becomes a millionaire overnight teaching people how to lose weight by eating just doughnuts.

How can this be you ask? This diet defies conventional wisdom. Or does it? How much calories are in a doughnut? Let's say there were 600 kcals in one of these doughnuts. So if you are eating one of these three times a day and that's all you are consuming, how many calories are you taking in, 1800 kcals right? That is how this gentleman is losing tons of weight. He is taking in fewer calories than his body requires to run. So his body has to burn its fat supply to run normally.

Is this person malnourished, you betcha. He is severely deficient in vitamins, minerals, and proteins. But remember he was malnourished to begin with, but now he is getting rid of all his disease causing fat. So he is still malnourished but he is at less risk of health complications from being at a healthy weight.

Please, please, please, know that I am not suggesting that anybody only eat doughnuts. I just like this illustration to hit home on the power of eating appropriate portions to lose weight.

So without further ado, I now introduce to you Phase 1 of the Fist Diet:

Eat the exact same way you are eating now, just less. Eat fist sized portions of calorie containing foods three times a day. **Fist size portions are only for the calorie containing foods.**

Your fist dimensions are not an exact science, use good judgment. Sure if you want to, you can figure out the exact mass of your fist and measure every meal accordingly. I say that jokingly; try not to over think it.

No calorie containing snacks. This might be the most difficult part of the Fist Diet for some of you out there; you can snack all you want however, the snacks just have to be zero or negative calorie. No calorie containing snacks.

Drink exactly whatever you are drinking now, just less. Drink half as much calorie containing amounts as you used to. Drink lots of water, as much as you can consume comfortably. Remember you are eating less not drinking less. It is important to avoid dehydration. Plus, drinking lots of water will help you feel full.

If you remember your motivation you will have the motivation to do this. If you follow phase 1 you should lose approximately 2-3 pounds a week. If you cheat by eating more than a fist sized portion of calorie containing foods per meal, by snacking on calorie containing food, or by drinking too much calorie containing drinks, you may only maintain your current weight or only lose one pound per week.

Phase 2 (Weight Loss and Health)

Eat less quantity and better quality foods. For Phase 1 you didn't change what you ate you just changed how much of it you ate (remember the doughnut dude). For Phase 2 we start to clean up what we are eating. Some of you will not have to even go into Phase 2 of the Fist Diet. If all you are trying to do is lose 10-30 pounds phase 1 will accomplish that for you. For those of us that plateau on phase 1 and we still want to lose weight, then we will have to move into phase 2.

For an example, in Phase 1 let's say you were eating just one fast food sausage muffin or burrito instead of three like normal. In Phase 2 you would skip the sausage muffin and eat a couple of hard boiled eggs or two of the small packages of Greek yogurt instead.

The sausage muffin is highly processed and will metabolize super-fast spewing fat and sugar into your blood stream immediately. The hard boiled eggs and yogurt on the other hand, will digest more slowly helping you to stay full longer to sustain you. The eggs/yogurt will not spike your blood sugar and all the protein in there will push hunger away a lot longer than the muffin.

In Phase 2 you will still eat fist sized portions of calorie containing foods three times a day. One of the big differences is that you will be eating nutrient dense and fewer processed foods. Remember, fist size portions are only for the calorie containing foods.

Again the fist sizing is not an exact science, use good judgment.

The other big difference between Phase 1 and 2 is that in Phase 2 you only consume very little to zero calories a day from beverages. You still need to drink lots of water, as much as you can consume comfortably making sure to avoid dehydration.

Sometimes we can drink more calories than we eat. Drink more water than you ever have in your life. This will help you to feel full and keep you healthy. Just because you are limiting your calorie intake does not mean that you are limiting your water intake.

Consume more fruits and vegetables than anything else; these are usually zero or negative calories thus making them free foods that you can eat as much of them as you want. Eating fruits and vegetables will ensure you are getting enough vitamins, minerals, content, and water.

Eat protein rich foods to be able to maintain and build muscle. Eating protein rich foods will help you to eat less at future meals. Examples include: Greek yogurt, eggs, lean meats, beans, and nuts.

Avoid simple carbs like white bread, chips and candy. These foods turn immediately into sugar once digested. Never look at a bun the same, from now on look at a piece of white bread or a hamburger bun as a cup of sugar.

Eat small amounts of complex carbohydrates, this will help you burn fat better and avoid burning lean muscles for the sugar stored in them.

Avoid the bad fats (LDL) and eat a small amount of the good fats.

Don't worry about the classifications of foods we will cover them in detail shortly.

Phase 3 (Health and Shape)

It's basically Phase 2 with a cuss word added:

Exercise

Exercise will help you reshape your body, decrease appetite, sharpen your mind, decrease your stress levels, help you sleep better, increase bone strength, increase immunity, lower cancer risks, strengthen lungs, heart, and vessels, lower risk of developing diabetes, reduce anxiety and depression, create a better self-image, and longer and higher quality of life, oh yeah and better sex life too.

However, you can lose lots of weight without ever exercising one bit. Phase 1 and 2 of the Fist Diet will knock off an easy 40- 50 pounds in 6 months. I lost a ton of weight but I still was not at my ideal shape. Once you lose most of your body fat it doesn't take much strength training to see fast results. I lifted weights off and on most of my life and never had great results. Once I got rid of my excess fat it was easier to see my muscles. Here I thought for all these years that you needed to pump iron nonstop to get cut. In reality all you need to do is to eradicate the excess fat to see the muscles and do minimal strength training.

You will speed up your weight loss with exercise. Exercise is also necessary for re-shaping your body. If you are going for a certain body shape and not just weight loss then be mentally prepared to exercise.

Exercising can be the most unpleasant thing we ever do. It can be fun too if we tie it into our passions. I really enjoy kick boxing so I got a free standing water filled punching bag. It's fun to beat on it and I am strength training and doing cardio while releasing frustration. If you love to rock climb, play the Wii, paintball, hunt, window shop, landscape photography then make time for it. All those things are exercise.

Exercise is more sustainable the more convenient we make it. Do it during TV time in your living room. Punch out a bunch of pushups during commercials.

Out of sight out of mind, where is your workout equipment? Put your treadmill in the living room and use as you watch TV. What do you want more a rocking body or a normal living room? Normal is not only overrated but it is inside the box and boring.

Exercising reduces your appetite. Diet pills can do the same, however diet pills won't do all the other things that exercise can: Heart health, burn calories, increase blood flow, etc.... Diet pills can be addictive and negatively interact with your essential medicines.

If you want muscle growth for looks, blood sugar control, improved work capacity, rehab from injury, etc... , break your previous work out records often; this will cause your body to break down and rebuild your muscle every time to meet the new demands (muscle growth). Don't get into a workout routine. Push yourself every time. Even if it is only one more rep or extra quarter lap. Change up the dates and times you do certain exercises. Cause your muscles to keep guessing and stay prepped for whatever. Do not give them a chance to get dormant.

When you feel terrible and depressed just do your favorite exercise. Even if you did it two days ago. As long as you have a day of rest in-between to rebuild, you can repeat the same exercise. When my workout motivation suffers I remind myself of my motivations to get healthy and when that is weak I just do my favorite work out at the time. Most often it is bench presses, pushups, heavy bag work, or jumping on the trampoline with my kids.

Exercising (Aerobic)

Exercises that require oxygen:

Fast walking, jogging, trampoline, kick boxing, etc... These types of exercises will burn the most fat if done at moderate intensity for over 20 min. The first 20 minutes your body just uses up its storages of sugar (glycogen) in your muscles. After that your body burns fat for energy. So if you are walking for 20 minutes every day then you are only eating up the sugar stored in your muscles. You might not have burned any fat at all. You did make a sugar vacuum in your muscles so when you do eat the sugars will be sucked into your muscles instead of converted to fat. So if 20 minutes is all you got than it is better than nothing. But if you want to burn mass amounts of fat then you got to do it longer. Walk fast enough where you are unable to sing. Don't walk so slow that you can sing effortlessly. If you can sing that dumb commercials jingle that's stuck in your head then its time to pick up the pace. You do not have to go so fast that you can't talk however. Just to the point where you need to focus on breathing.

If you are able to jog or run, then walk a fast lap and jog a slow lap for 45 min. This will burn a ton of fat. If you can run the whole time great, but if you can't then walking fast in-between jogging laps will keep your heart rate up enough to get the intended effect.

Exercising (Anaerobic)

Exercises that don't require oxygen are anaerobic:

Lifting weights, offensive/defensive line, pushups, lunges, squats, etc... These exercises are powered by the sugar (glycogen) stored in your muscles already.

However, they build muscle which loves to eat sugar, so the calories you consume from carbohydrates will be taken up by your muscles and not turned into fat.

Muscles rule. They will make you look younger, work harder, play more, and feel great. If you are a guy, a good rule of thumb to look good is to have your pecks stick out farther then your belly and have some bulk in your arms. If you are a chick, then you want definition. Don't focus on low reps of heavy weights. If you do this you will look like a dude from far away. Instead, focus on light weights and mass reps, this will give your muscles a long smooth and defined look.

Work Out Routines

If you are on Phase 3 of the Fist Diet, then it is time to a work out.

Two to three times a week is average, once a week is not enough, every day may be excessive.

Don't let your body get used to your routine, switch it up. Having a diverse plan will keep you from getting bored as well. Set goals, slaughter them and set new ones.

Give muscle groups at least a day of rest before you hit it again. You don't have to work out for hours on end, try doing just one thing a day three times a week to start. If you start off going crazy you might burn yourself out.

Knowing that you have a three hour workout planned for tonight will take more mental preparation/motivation than knowing all you have to do is push-ups. However if you are motivated enough and you want to work out every day, make sure you are not doing the same muscle groups consecutively. You may be doing a different move or activity but they both may use the same muscle group.

Make a spread sheet. A spread sheet will help you track what you are doing, when you are doing it, and how much of it you are doing. Put all the workout moves you will actually do on it. If you are not going to do clapping push-ups then skip them on your list. Track stuff like: date, time, repetitions, weight, sets, distance, and duration.

Work out at work, when your super slow computer is booting up, when you are waiting for something to load, or at break time. All these situations are great for dropping to the floor and doing some push-ups, sit ups, lunges, etc...

Force Your Body To Burn Fat To Survive

If your body wants to survive make it burn all the stored fat for energy. It won't be happy, but it is not in charge. We are in charge and we are motivated to lose weight. We made a decision to change our lifestyle and body shape.

There is 3500 calories in one pound of fat. That is a lot of energy. I lost 60 pounds, so that means I had eaten 210,000 more calories than I needed to function normally. That's 1312.5 12 oz. pops/sodas, that is 291 Whoppers.

Most diets focus on what you can or cannot eat. They miss the simple truth. If you consume fewer calories than you burn you will lose weight. It doesn't matter if you are eating their prepackaged foods or from the gas station. You have enough stored energy to power yourself though the day. Eating fist sized portions of calorie containing foods, zero and negative calorie foods will make sure you are getting enough content for your gastrointestinal tract function and making sure your get enough essential nutrients that aren't found in fats. Also you need to eat some carbs just to burn fats effectively without sending your body into a state of ketosis. Diets that make you eliminate carbs will cause you to lose weight by breaking down your muscles for the sugar in them and these diets will cause ketosis to develop in your blood stream due to the absence of carbohydrates.

How Many Calories Can I Ingest?

This is a very debated and hot topic. The short answer is specific to each person. It depends on a lot of variables like age, sex, muscles mass, weight, and activity level. It is not recommended to go under 800 calories a day. Could you eat 2000 kcals a day and lose weight? Sure, depending on the variables.

Those with the DNA and genes that make them tall and stout will need more calories than those who are naturally vertically challenged.

The Fist Diet is designed to make, or force your body to burn all its excess fat for fuel. You can do this by doing a moderate exercise for over 20 minutes. Or by simply ingesting fewer calories than your body requires. When you take in fewer calories than your body requires, it has to get fuel from somewhere. Where does it find the fuel? Well it just so happens that your body was designed with roll over minutes. When we eat more calories than we burn the extra goes into storage. This is called fat. So when you eat only fist sized portions of calorie containing foods three times a day your body will tap into that storage supply for this rainy day. Now when your body does this every day for several months your reserve supplies will start to dry up. Wha la you are now free from excess body fat. It's time now to up your intake a little to maintain your ideal weight.

The Fist Diet is also designed to give us our lives back from obsessing over diet rules and counting. How many calories are in that? How many points is that worth? If I eat this what would be my options for dinner?

With the Fist Diet phase 1 it's not about what you eat it's about how much of it you eat. It's time to take back our mind's time and give our mental powers to more important things than diet dos and don'ts.

No Calories From Snacks

We are all guilty of falling victim to the snack attack. Sometimes we can eat as much or more calories with our snacks as we do with our meals. Snacking is not bad however, snacking on bad things is. For all three phases of the Fist Diet it is important to not snack on any calorie containing foods. You can eat all the zero and negative calories foods you want however.

Every calorie containing snack you eat will take away from your body's need to burn your excess fat for fuel. So if you decide to snack on calorie containing foods you will slow down your progress.

Are you an all-day snacker? Do you eat constantly all day instead of eating meals?

I know several people who fit into this category. If we do this we will have a difficult time figuring out how many calories we ingested, total portions, how much protein, fat, and carbs we took in.

So what am I saying? It would be a lot easier to lose weight if we only ate three meals a day. Now if this is impossible for you then try this. Keep eating all day but cut your snacks in half. Keep drinking calorie containing beverages all day but cut the amount you drink in half. If you are not losing weight fast enough then cut out all your calorie containing drinks and switch to zero kcal drinks. If you are still not losing weight fast enough then cut your snack portions down further. If all this fails quit snacking all day and move into the three meals a day routine. Most of the snack all day folks are not eating that way because of a health reason, it usually boils down to not taking the time to sit down and eat.

Favorite Unhealthy Foods

Go ahead and eat your favorite unhealthy foods every now and then. Just eat it in your fist size. If you think this sounds too good to be true you are right. The catch is that you will have to substitute it for a meal. If you are in Phase 1 you can eat whatever you want already just in fist sized portions three times a day. If you are in Phase 2 you should be eating cleaner burning, less processed more natural and nutrient dense foods. Your favorite unhealthy foods probably do not fit into this category. But you can still indulge yourself with these foods in Phase 2 or 3 just do it infrequently and in fist size.

Favorite Unhealthy Drinks

Phase 1: Keep drinking them just cut your intake by 50-75%.

Phase 2: Go ahead and drink your favorite unhealthy drink every now and then. If it contains too many calories then to stay on track you will have to substitute it for a meal. This is not recommended due to malnourishment issues, however in moderation it will be OK.

Phase 3: Same as phase two.

Energy Source Transition Period (Mutiny)

When you reach the point where your body has to actually burn fat for energy, it will start to rebel even more. Your body will act like it is dying to try to get you to return to obeyig it and overeat. This will have a mental/physical effect on you and will cause you to second guess yourself. Steady the course. Don't listen to your flesh. It has gotten you to the weight you are, why would we go back to obeying it? The flesh just wants to have fun. It does not care about the consequences. It does not care about your waist line. It's time to impeach and dethrone it and take our life back.

Hunger pangs caused from changing to smaller portions will go away.

If you can't calm yourself down with logic then do the following:

Switch to Phase 2 and eat better food that is more nutrient dense. Get more rest. Drink more water. If the mutiny lasts for more than a week after you have tried these, then increase calorie intake a little.

3 Months later

You lost 30-40 pounds and you still don't have the shape you are going for, and if a specific shape is more important to you than a specific weight, it may be time to start Phase 3: Cardio and strength training.

You are at your ideal weight. Now what? Don't stop eating healthy and appropriate portions. Now it's maintenance time. Maintaining is a lot easier than losing. Continue to weigh and/or measure once a week and adjust your intake to maintain your ideal weight or shape.

You will probably have to increase your intake a little to stop losing weight.

Plateauing

To plateau is normal.

Once you change your eating habits to only a fist sized portion of calorie containing foods per meal three times a day you might stop losing weight by that alone. You may then need to clean up what you are eating a fist size of and move to Phase 2. Or worst case scenario, you might have to add a little exercising to your routine and jump into Phase 3.

1 Year Later

You will enter a cycle where you become depressed and frustrated. A death, job loss, breakup, or any other countless negative situations might occur. Plan for them and don't turn to food to cope. It will be easy to forget your motivation once you have accomplished your goal. It is important during these trying times to remember your motivating factors.

Maintenance

Once you achieve your ideal weight and body shape you will have undoubtedly formed a fist sized eating habit. To maintain weight you will need to increase your portions slightly. If you continue eating only fist sized portions you will continue to lose weight. If you were eating two eggs for breakfast and two cups of Greek yogurt for lunch try adding one more egg or cup of yogurt to your meal. During your weekly weigh in you will be able to monitor if you are consuming enough to maintain your weight rather than gain or lose. If increasing your breakfast and lunch portions is causing a slight weight gain than just increase one of your meal's portions rather than both of them.

Bad Craving Cycle

As humans we go through different mental cycles in our lives. While you are going through a really bad craving cycle of worthless foods it's OK to switch to Phase 1 until the cycle is over. Remember you can lose weight eating junk as long as it is in fist sized portions and only three times a day. This will lead to malnourishment if you do this for too long. But, substituting a well-balanced meal for a slice of pie is OK as long as it is not for every meal for a week straight. Again, this is the sustainable beauty of the Fist Diet. Pie is not evil; no food is off limits and evil. We just stop abusing/misusing it and don't overeat it anymore.

Breakfast

You must have it. Skipping breakfast will cause you to overeat at lunch and dinner. Skipping breakfast is used as a justification to overeat at later meals. Keep it simple, high protein, convenient and fast. Once a week hard boil 12-18 eggs, peel and bag two to three in each bag. Grab a bag everyday as you head out the door. You can eat these on the go. Eggs are in high protein, super low in simple carbs, and contain enough fat to sustain and satisfy you. Plus they only contain about 80 calories per egg.

Eating breakfast will keep the hunger pangs and stomach noises away. When lunch time comes, you wont be chomping at the bit to beat down a burger.

Lunch

Before the Fist Diet, an hour for lunch was not enough. Now you will have extra time for yourself. When you order your meal get it to go even if you are sitting in. Your lunch in the past was barely enough to satisfy; now it will last for two to three lunches.

If you are packing a lunch; eat some Greek Yogurt, or homemade burritos. Remember, we are only eating enough to last us until dinner not until December.

If work is super stressful and you have to munch for your sanity; bring some baby carrots or celery. All the crunching will help you cope with the stress. Exercising is also a great alternative to snacking for stress. We need to break the cycle that food is an anti-stress medication. In your office do some pushups, crunches, lunges, or squats. Not enough to get all sweaty, but enough to get some positive endorphins going to relieve stress. Take your stress out on the floor with pushups instead of taking it out on your digestive system.

Dinner

Now is the time for an elaborate meal. Only ingest a calorie containing food the size of your fist. However, you can eat a mountain of zero or negative calorie foods if you want to. Eat slowly, take a half time, and keep the TV and computer off during meal times.

We should never eat when we are distracted. If we mentally focus on our meal we will know that we ate. Have you ever eaten chips while you were watching TV? After a couples hours on the couch the bag of chips is empty and we barely remember eating all of them. That is because we weren't focused on eating them. If we were eating the bag of chips with the TV off, we would not have eaten the entire bag.

Here is a loophole to eat a plateful of food and a mealtime; if you are cooking for one, use a fist size amount of calorie containing foods with a ton of zero or negative calorie foods. When you go to "plate it", your plate will be full, however you will only be consuming a fist size of calorie containing foods per plate. For example: take a ¼ pound of ground beef and cook it with a mountain of sliced up bell peppers, onions, and tomatoes.

Home Cooking

Not Rocket Surgery; with the birth of the microwave and when we started Idolizing chefs in the 70s came the demise of the home cook. The average American believes that cooking something other than macaroni and cheese is too difficult and that they don't have the skills to pull it off. We have been programmed that we have to have a degree in culinary arts in order to cook something on the stove top or in the oven.

Home cooking is one of the pleasures in life we are missing out on. Think about it. You can make whatever you want, whenever you want, however you want it. What other time in life do we have that much freedom, power and creative control?

Not only is it fun but it is cost effective. You can make breakfast and lunch for your whole work week with the same amount of money as going out for lunch two times.

It is also a lot healthier. Not only are the hairs and germs in the food yours but you are eating less processed foods with fewer preservatives. Think about the food at restaurants; it was made by machines a month or two ago. It traveled across the county in a semi-truck, and is reheated by a dude with more metal in his face than Dick Chaney's hunting partner. To get food to keep that long the industrial food manufactures have to add a lot of chemical preservatives. I know some of you out there think that by consuming preservatives it will preserve you and make you live longer but odds are it will probably just give you cancer.

Cooking at home is a wonderful creative outlet. Don't just slop it on a plate. Actually plate it. Make it look pretty. Remember we eat with our eyes and mind just as much as with our taste buds.

I can give the same meal to two different people. Plate one pretty and slop the other on a paper plate and they will give two different reviews about the same tasting food.

Cook outside the box. Don't get caught up in the fact that you never heard of those ingredients in the same meal before. If you like them both then give it a try. Who knows, you might invent the next big thing in food.

Just open your fridge throw all of your left overs in to a baking pan, top it with some cheese and bake it.

If you want to cut calories but still get a meaty flavor use meat as a seasoning instead of as the main attraction. You would be amazed how much beef flavor you will get out of a 1/16 pound of ground beef. Also, use veggies as noodles. This trick will decrease your calorie intake from carbs tremendously while still giving you the bulk you are used to ingesting.

Home cooking is healthier, fun, safer, cheaper, more gratifying, and tastes better than eating out. It also can produce self-esteem and help you unwind from the negativity you faced at work all day.

"Go-To" Ingredients

Bragg's Liquid Amino Soy Sauce

This is one of my favorite seasonings. It is loaded with flavor, contains zero calories, and it takes steamed veggies and stir-fry's to a restaurant quality level.

Made from Soy bean protein

Less salt than regular soy sauce

Great for stir fry, rice or any time you want a soy sauce or salty flavor

Dice up every vegetable in your refrigerator

Add some oil into a sauce pan

Sautee the veggies until desired softness

Season with Brag

You can consume a mountain of this without adding to the waistline or sacrificing flavor.

Special K Chips

Tastes like potatoes chips

Made from potatoes

You can eat 30 for only 110 calories

Great with hummus, salsa, queso con carne dip, or for anything you would have used regular chips.

Couch Time

This still is the most difficult time of day for me to stick to the plan. After a hard day of work when I finally make it home, I eat a mountain of steamed or stir fried veggies with a fist size of calorie containing food on the side. Then move to the couch for some much needed rest. After about an hour or two I want to eat a snack.

Eating while you watch TV is an American tradition that dates back to the birth of the television. We Americans grew up doing it and still do it every night we can. Eating while we watch TV is also a contributing factor in America's obesity problem. Have you heard the term "couch potato"?

Here are some Fist Diet strategies to overcome this deeply ingrained enemy of the waste line tradition:

Go with it. But switch up what you are ingesting, eating all the zero or negative calorie snacks you want instead.

Logically go through your day and remind yourself of the awesome nutritious food you have eaten for breakfast, lunch and dinner (Phase 2 & 3). Or at least remind yourself that the small fist size meals of bad food still gave you adequate calories for the day (Phase 1).

Work out instead of eating while you watch TV, do paperwork, go through mail, and keep your mind occupied.

Most importantly, remember your motivation for losing weight. Remember all the reasons you are denying your flesh. Remember why you took control over your carnal desires and waged a war on your cravings to begin with. If these reasons are still what you want, you will be able to overcome your cravings.

If at any time you decide you want to eat whatever you want, whenever you want, more than you want to live healthy and happy than you will lose this battle.

Here is a sample daily diet plan for Phase 1 of the Fist Diet. The point of this sample is to show that you could eat anything you want in a fist portion and still lose weight.

Sample Diet Phase 1

Breakfast:

One or two small breakfast burritos

Black coffee or water to drink

Lunch:

Small cheese burger

Diet pop, unsweetened ice tea or water to drink

Dinner:

A mountain of steamed veggies and a fist sized portion of chicken, beef, turkey, pork, tofu, beans and rice, pasta and sauce, or whatever calorie containing food you want like; one slice of pizza or one piece of pie.

Now, depending on what you eat you may not be getting the nutrients your body needs to perform at maximum. Having said that, Phase 1 is a great way to lose weight with as little change as possible. If you eat fast food for all three of your meals, you can still do that. You will continue to be malnourished but at least now you are losing lots of disease causing fat.

Here are two sample diets for Phase 2 of the Fist Diet. Remember in Phase 2 we are still only eating fist sized portions of calorie containing foods three times a day. The big change from Phase 1 and Phase 2 is that we are cleaning up what we eat. We are consuming mostly nutrient dense and protein rich foods.

Sample Diet Phase 2

Breakfast: Two cups of Greek Yogurt with coffee or water to drink

Lunch: One medium to large chicken breast with diet pop, water, or unsweetened iced tea to drink

Dinner: A mountain of steamed veggies and a fist size amount of a protein rich food

Sample Diet Phase 2

Breakfast: Two slices of a an 15 egg frittata or two to three hard boiled eggs with black coffee or water to drink

Lunch: One or two homemade burritos on small flour tortillas and diet pop, water, or unsweetened iced tea to drink

Dinner: A plateful of stir fried veggies with nuts and a 1/8 pound of ground beef and diet pop, water, or unsweetened iced tea to drink

Vacation

Vacation time = party time right? No work, no deadlines, no problems. It's time to let loose, chill and do something really fun.

Who on earth would diet on a vacation? Who would want to bring that vibe into a let loose environment?

The answer is anyone who is trying to reach their ideal shape and weight. Here are some strategies to stick to the plan without becoming a major buzz kill to your family on your vacation.

If you were on Phase 2 or 3 of the Fist Diet you could pack a whole bunch of nutrient dense foods with you and put them in the hotel's little room refrigerator. You could try to order protein rich foods at whatever restaurant you are eating. Or you could just switch to Phase 1 for your vacation.

That means that you just go with the flow and eat wherever the rest of the family is eating whenever the family is eating. You can order whatever you want on the menu and just eat a fist sized portion of it and save the little hotel fridge for all your killer leftovers.

Once you get back home and into your routine you can go back to Phase 2 or 3.

Fist Travel Tips

I don't know about you, but when I travel I like to eat the whole time. Eating keeps me awake and it offers me some pleasure while doing something I'd rather not be doing. If you are eating snacks from the gas station each time you fill up, not only will your wallet lose weight, but you will gain weight. When we are traveling we are not burning as many calories, and to consume 2000-4000, that day from road food and snacks will surely result in a higher intake to calorie burn ratio, meaning we will pick up some extra pounds.

Here is an alternative; Pack negative calorie fruits and vegetables for your trip. Wash and bag a ton of baby carrots and apples. Chow on them during your drive instead of a pastry, bag of chips, or a candy bar.

Sometimes if I am on an all-day drive, I will skip a meal and just snack healthy the entire trip.

If you have to purchase your snacks at the gas station go for the healthy nut mixes and fruit. More and more gas stations are stocking their shelves with fruit. Also grab a few pickles while you are there. They are zero calorie and take a while to eat. Rip the bag open on the way to your car, dump out the juice in the trash can and eat down the road.

Holidays

It is impossible to celebrate a holiday without a ton of food involved. This year for Thanksgiving I will go to four huge dinners consecutively. I'll start with a church Thanksgiving dinner on Tuesday, a work Thanksgiving potluck on Wednesday, Thursday we'll do the wife's side of the family dinner, ending the week with a Friday my side of the family's Thanksgiving dinner. Oh yea I forgot to mention the left overs that will be overloading our fridge.

What's a guy to do that's trying to maintain or lose weight?

Easy, remember your motivation and reasons. Read them out loud every day. Ponder them; remember why they are important to you. After doing that it will be easier to not over eat. Because achieving your goals will give you long lasting rewards that will trump any pumpkin pie. Remember you can eat whatever you want to for three meals a day just do it in fist sized portions. So you won't have to miss out on your aunt's corn bread stuffing or your mom's special pies.

Here is another strategy; I use this one when I get roped into going to buffets too. Only put the best of the best on your plate. If you don't like your sister in laws mashed potatoes and gravy then don't put it on your plate. You can only eat so much so don't waste it on bland or dry food.

Load up on the veggie platter. Trust me there will be plenty left. You may be the only person eating them. Get full on celery and cauliflower and top it off with a fist size of the best of the best.

You can survive this holiday and stay on track. Food does not have a remote control to your brain. If you want to reach your ideal weight/body shape bad enough then you will.

Besides this holiday is supposed to be about thinking of all the many blessings we have, not about eating until we feel sick. So let us be thankful for our lives instead of damaging our lives due to the negative mental and physical effects of overeating.

Dining Out

When you order your meal get it to go even if you are sitting in, or ask for a to go box as soon as you get your food. Keep a fist size portion of food on your plate and put the rest in the container. Your friends will make fun of you but will soon shut up when you are rocking your new look. Avoid buffets if you can, or eat a mountain of zero/negative calorie foods there so we can feel we got our money's worth.

Eat Slowly

When we eat slowly at the restaurant we won't feel funny that we are done first and are staring at everyone else eating. I know we should not have to do these kinds of tricks to avoid persecution for our new lifestyle change. But odds are you will not get praised for eating appropriate portions but rather ridiculed. Your new lifestyle change (diet) will cause conviction in everyone around. Most of them will give you some kind of negative remarks.

Trust me it is worth the social persecution from 99% of the people in your life to get healthy. They will stop messing with you once they are used to your new shape. For me it took everyone about six months to stop making negative comments. After a while it isn't news anymore and people will stop "player hating" you.

Artificial Sweetener Overdosing

 New artificial sweeteners are popping up on the market almost every day and in new products, We could spend a day or two meticulously contemplating the pros and cons of each one. I don't spend much time on the subject because it mostly matters if you are trying to choose an artificial sweetener to buy to use as an ingredient. If I am making something I need to be sweet I will use brown sugar or honey. I'm only going to consume a fist sized portion of it anyway so I might as well enjoy the real deal and taste. Plus I already ingest too much of this stuff in my beverages.

Food manufactures switched to this stuff for the marketability of a product with "no sugar added" and one with "low carbs". They also can get these chemical concoctions for a lot less than real sugar. So far the new studies out show these products to be safe and nonharmful, but I will let you know if I start growing a third arm. I do consume a lot of these products like everyone else who is eating prepared food from the store. However, I try to limit my intake to just what I get from diet pop. You will find artificial sweeteners in yogurt, diet pop, candy, and any other premade foods that formerly had sugar as an ingredient. It's OK to ingest a small amount of fake sugar, just don't live off the stuff.

While we are talking about fake sugar let me take this opportunity to say something about food with real sugar in it. "No sugar added" does not mean no sugar ingested. You will see many products with the slogan on their labels "no sugar added". Flip it over to the back a guess what? You will usually see lots of sugars or carbs listed in the nutrition facts. I noticed this again at Thanksgiving time. I was told a pie was "sugar free", but in fact it was just "no sugar added". The store bought pie filling boasted the label "no sugar added" and were telling the truth. However, the product was loaded with carbs. How can this be? The ingredients had their own sugars naturally and the manufacturers didn't add any more. So the next time you hear the phrase "no sugar added", remember that it does not mean no sugar ingested.

Sugar free does not mean calorie free; even if a product naturally does not contain sugar and has not had any sugar added to it, it does not mean that it is calorie free. Calories come from a lot of different sources. Actually fat contains more calories per gram than sugar. So if you are watching your calorie intake be careful to not overindulge in a product labeled "sugar free", because "sugar free" or "low carb" does not mean no or low calories. A hot dog can be sugar free but is has enough calories to run the car from the Back to the Future movies for a week.

Negative Calorie Vegetables

Here are some negative calorie vegetables: asparagus, beet root, broccoli, cabbage, carrot, cauliflower, celery chicory, hot chili, cucumber, garden cress, garlic, green beans, lettuce, onion, radish, spinach, turnip, and zucchini.

But there are only really a handful of veggies we should consume in fist sized portions. Most veggies will not affect your waistline and you can get full all day on them without causing a depressing scale moment. The veggies on my fist portion list are: corn, potatoes, and sweet potatoes. Some negative calorie gurus will argue with me on this but I lost a ton of weight eating a ton of veggies that were not on their negative calorie lists.

The catch to enjoying a ton of these vegetables without tipping your calorie ingested vs. burned ratio, is that you cannot add calories to these when you eat them. So if you just beat down a huge bowl of celery but you dipped each one in ranch then you ingested a lot of calories. Or if you steam up a mountain of these bad boys but added a mountain of butter to them, then you are in the high calorie range.

So steam them up but season with just salt and pepper or one of my favorite ways to enjoy them is with some bragg soy sauce.

Negative Calorie Fruits

Here is a list of some negative calorie fruits: apple, blueberry, cantaloupe, cranberry, grapefruit, honeydew, lemon/lime, mango, orange, papaya, peach, pineapple, raspberry, strawberry, tomato, tangerine, and watermelon.

Carbohydrates

Carbs contain four calories per gram. Most everything our bodies need for energy in carbs can be obtained from burning fat. Go ahead and eat them, but only in fist size. Avoid simple carbs like: chips, candy, and pastries. Simple carbs break down extremely fast; this causes a jump in blood sugar and a higher conversion to fat risk.

Chose complex carbs like: whole grain breads, wild rice, certain veggies. These also bring with them a load of fiber and take longer for your body to break them down. Our body does need carbs. Our brain, nerves and to make new red blood cells which require the energy from carbs. If we cut out carbs completely, our body will tear down lean muscle to get the sugar inside them to sustain brain function. Also to burn fat more efficiently, we need some carbs available in our system to avoid excessive ketone accumulation in the blood (ketosis).

Fat

Why does our bodies make and store fat? What is fat?

Fats contain 9 calories per gram and is an awesome source of energy. A fat cell is comprised of 80% fat, 18% water, and 2% protein. Fat cells can also contain a small amount of glycogen. Fat (adipose tissue) has a high turnover rate. The belly fat you saw today is completely different then the belly fat you saw a month ago. So the more fat you have, the more stored energy you have. Fat also stores toxins DDT, PCB, etc....

There is a lot of research out there that suggests that burning your body fat instead of burning ingested food for energy causes an increase in mental acuity, energy, and other benefits to your brain.

There are good fats and bad fats; (HDL) High Density Lipoproteins: These are the good kinds of fats that remove cholesterol from your body, (LDL) Low Density Lipoproteins: Raise cholesterol levels and thus increase risk for heart diseases.

(LDL) Low Density Lipoproteins

Sources: LDLs are mainly found in trans fatty acids that come from animal products and foods with a long shelf life. Trans fatty acids preservatives were invented in 1890. Eating less processed foods and animal products will reduce your LDLs.

(HDL) High Density Lipoproteins

Sources: HDLs are found in unsaturated vegetable oils from canola, peanuts, olive, flax, corn, safflower and sunflower. They are also found in avocados, nuts, and salmon. Eating these foods regularly will decrease your chances of heart trouble.

Protein

Proteins contain 4 calories per gram. Proteins rule. Proteins are building blocks for muscles, and muscles burn calories even at rest. Muscles are good: for looks, posture, weight maintenance, and the ability to work harder without injury. Your calorie intake for the day should mainly come from proteins.

Alcohol

Alcohol contains 7 calories per gram. Do you have a beer belly or a pony keg?

Vitamins, Minerals, and Supplements

It is recommended if you are on Phase 1 to take a multivitamin. During Phase 1 you can eat whatever you want just in fist sizes. For those of us that will take full nutritional naughty advantage of this dietary freedom, we may not be meeting our nutritional needs. If you decide to take a multivitamin it is a great idea to also take some probiotics. You may not be metabolizing your supplements if your digestive track is clogged. If you are on Phase 2, you probably do not need to take them at all. If you are eating nutrient dense whole foods chances are you are getting plenty of vitamins naturally, especially if you are consuming a mountain of steamed veggies every night.

Vitamins and minerals are essential to sustain our lives. We need to consume and digest them as much as possible. The best source for them is in food not in pills. A lot of foods that are high in these are also zero or negative calorie foods.

Digestive Health

All of the over processed fake plastic food we have been eating for years has clogged or digestive tracts. If our digestive tract is clogged, we will be unable to absorb the nutrients in the foods we eat.

Probiotics are actually live, good bacteria that will eat everything in your digestive system that doesn't belong. They will keep your G.I. system clean and clear so you can absorb all the nutrients and water from your food. You could take an over the counter probiotic but I prefer to just eat Greek yogurt or drink some Kefir.

Glycemic Index

Some foods will turn to sugar faster than others. This is bad for diabetics and those losing weight. We want to eat foods that take a long time to break down, thus giving our body time to burn off the calories before they get turned into fat. Usually processed foods are the fastest to turn into sugar then into fat. The less processed the food the longer it will take our body to break it down. It's like throwing some particle board on a fire, that wood is compressed and glued together. It will burn hot and fast. If you throw actual logs on the fire they will burn for hours. A hamburger is the particle board and beans and brown rice would be the log.

Body Mass Index

Body Mass Index (B.M.I.) is a number calculated from a person's height and weight. B.M.I. is one useful tool to test appropriate fat ratio. The downfall of the B.M.I. is that it does not take into account lots of muscle mass or a severe lack of muscle mass.

To calculate your body mass index: Multiply your weight in pounds by 703. Then divide that number by your height in inches squared.

Example: 170 lbs. x 703 = 119510 65

Inches squared = 4225

119510/4225 = 28.28

28.28 is your B.M.I.

BMI Categories:

•Underweight = <18.5

•Normal weight = 18.5–24.9

•Overweight = 25–29.9

•Obesity = BMI of 30 or greater

Body Fat Percentage

Body fat percentage is measured by dividing your total weight by the weight of your fat. There are many different ways to measure your body fat. Two popular ways to measure are by bioelectrical impedance and by using a body fat caliper. These tools can range from $12.00 -$1000.00

Body Fat Percentage Chart

Description	Women	Men
Essential fat	8–12%	3–5%
Athletes	14-20%	6–13%
Fitness	21-24%	14–17%
Average	25-32%	18-24%
Excess fat	32%+	25%+

Sculpted/Defined/Ripped

Being sculpted is more about body fat percentage then it is about muscle mass. I have lifted a lot of weights in my life but never achieved a sculpted look. When I started the Fist Diet and started losing weight, I noticed that my muscles were popping out. When I started Phase 3 and started to hit the weights, it did not take long to get that sculpted physique. Amazing, my whole life I was trying to get a ripped look the wrong way, all I had to do was get rid of the excess body fat so my muscles could show their definition.

Professional body builders get down to 6-10% body fat for a competition. That is why we can see all their muscles. These same people during the off season have the same muscles but are not nearly as ripped because they pick up around 40 pounds of fat when not in competition. So if you want to get ripped, rip off the excess body fat. If you want to get sculpted, first let the Fist Diet sculpt off the love handles. And if you want to get defined, remove all the rounding agent otherwise known as fat.

Weighing

Weigh only once per week. Otherwise when you are on track and doing great you will discourage yourself. You are not going to lose so much weight that it will be noticeable every day. If you lose three pounds a week that is only 0.4285714 pounds a day, 0.4285714 pounds is not noticeable on most scales.

I like to use my kid's Wii balance board to weigh. It tracks, charts, and graphs my weigh-ins. I can see what I weighed when I first started and every week since. It allows you to set goals and does the math for you. It also calculates your B.M.I. and gives you your text book B.M.I. number.

Measuring

In addition to weighing or instead of weighing, you could measure your waist line. This will give you a different perspective on your weight loss. Some people will lose inches off their waistline but only lose small amounts of pounds. This too should still only be done once a week.

Measuring is also good if you are doing consistent strength training and dieting. You may be losing fat but staying at a steady weight. This may be a result of losing fat but gaining lean muscle mass. If you were to only weigh, it is possible to become discouraged with your progress. If you measure instead of weigh, you will be able to quantify your progress by a loss of waistline circumference.

Doctor

Listen to your Dr. if he/she tells you that due to your medical problems this lifestyle change would be too risky, then, you should heed their advice. However, it would be extremely rare for a physician to not advise you to eat less.

Married Folks

Substitute eating with something else pleasure producing, if you can't figure out anything else pleasure producing to do together, do the following: get alone with no distractions locked in your bedroom and I'm sure you can come up with something.

Be supportive. Do it together. Don't "player hate". Do it by yourself if you have to.

If the person who does the majority of the cooking refuses to hook you up with a mountain of steamed veggies every night with a side of fist sized calorie containing food, remember this; they may not want you to lose weight and look good due to their own insecurities. If this is the case we need to work on reassuring them of our love, commitment, and devotion to them. We should show this by words and deeds.

Consider also that we may have trained them that we will not stick to a new diet for more than a month. They might think that they should not even bother with this new plan because it won't last. If this is the case all we have to do is show them different through consistency. When they place a huge (normal) portion of calorie loaded food in front of you at dinner, just eat a fist size of it and then go eat some fruit on the couch. The message will be received if we are consistent. To be consistent all we have to do is take this one meal at a time and remember our motivation for losing weight.

If on the other hand you are the one that does most of the cooking and your spouse is not changing their eating habits with you, well it is an easier obstacle than the person in the above paragraph. Either cook and eat what they want but you eat it in fist size, or make your own meal different from theirs.

When you start losing weight and keeping it off you have just out done the best diet infomercial ever made. Your living example may in fact be what was needed to convince your spouse that they can do it too. So don't give up hope or degrade them for continuing to kill themselves with a spoon. Do the Fist Diet for yourself and you just might have support in your own house soon.

Family

Eat what everybody else is just less of it or make your plate different. There is an interesting phenomenon with kids however. It is the fact they believe that the food on your plate tastes better than the food on their plate even when it is the exact same food. Use this to your advantage and load up your plate with veggies and you may influence a child to develop healthy eating habits while they are young.

Back when I was not on the Fist Diet we would hit up the fast food joints for at least three family meals a week. My oldest daughter would only eat chicken nuggets. The most she would branch out was to eat chicken nuggets from a chain that didn't have a huge yellow M on it. My son and youngest daughter would only eat cheese roll ups, while my wife and I were content on eating several chicken and rice burritos.

Without trying we were training our kids that eating trash chain foods frequently is an acceptable practice. They were too young to correlate daddies and mommies extra weight with the unhealthy eating practices. If we were to continue on this trend they would grow up and have their parents body shapes. Do you have your parent's body shape and size when they were your age?

We had our work cut out for us because of these habits we had developed in our children. They still get to eat at the Yellow M store but only once a week. This way it is not harmful and is a real treat for them instead of being expected and not appreciated. It is also a lot better on my wallet too.

But due to their bad food start it has been challenging to recreate new palates and eating behaviors in them. We have succeeded in doing this but it took consistent healthy family meals for many months to get there.

My kids can all recognize several different vegetables and enjoy them without pitching a major fit.

You are eating less, not your kids. So while you may plate only a fist size portion for yourself, make sure they are getting enough good calories to grow. Also, at your family dinners keep the TV off and talk, this will be great for your family bonding and also help you to eat slow. Ask lots of questions, tell family stories, and have them tell you stories.

Diabetics

When you were first diagnosis with type 2 diabetes were you overwhelmed with the diet they told you to do from now on? Do you remember how foreign and complicated it was? Do you understand it any better now? Did you master counting carbs? Do you still count carbs? Do you still have type 2 diabetes?

If you get and stay on the Fist Diet, you can get rid of the disease altogether. You can quit counting carbs, and get off the meds that have all those nasty side effects. The average type two diabetic only has to lose 25-60 pounds for the disease to go away. You can do this in 2-5 months on the Fist Diet. Imagine going to the Doctor and having them tell you that your type two diabetes is gone and all you have to do to keep it gone is maintain your current weight.

Losing weight is as simple as finding the motivation and using it to make a decision at every meal to eat less.

Athletes

The Fist Diet is good for those trying to stay in a certain weight class or get fit enough to continue playing. Fat = weight which is hard on your joints. You may think you are too old to play that sport or hobby; however it may just be your weight and not your age at all.

Vegetarians

Vegetarians need to combine multiple foods to get enough amino acids to create proteins. This can cause them to eat larger meals. They can still do the Fist Diet, it will just take a little more meal planning to ensure adequate protein intake. This however is true for everyone.

Gluten Free

Gluten is a protein found in wheat. It is found as a thickening agent (dextrin) in ice cream, lip products, medications, and ketchup. It's used as flavoring and a food stabilizer. People with celiac disease, dermatitis herpetiformis, or a wheat allergy you will need to avoid it. As far as the Hollywood diet trend, just make sure you are getting enough fiber, foliate, and iron.

Lactose Intolerant

Blessing or Curse? While dairy products do contain lots of calcium and proteins they also contain lots of fat and cholesterol. So even though this group is missing out on the cheesy flavor, they are also missing out on the fat and cholesterol.

People who are lactose intolerant will have no problems with the Fist Diet in relation to their intolerance to the lactose found in dairy products.

Off Track

And? Get back on track. Don't beat yourself up and don't quit. Just fall off track less, and take less time to get back on track. You will lose the weight faster the more consistent you are, but having said that, you will never lose the weight if you beat yourself up and quit.

Consistency

Consistency is the name of the game. If we remember our motivation when we want to overeat, we will choose to accomplish our goal rather than to have seconds of pleasure followed by guilt. If we eat less and exercise consistently, we will achieve our goals.

Rocket Surgery

So the magic to loosing tons of weight is as simple as eating less, eating better, and staying active. This formula is tried, true and safe.

Morals of the Story

Phase 1: Eat Less.

Phase 2: Eat less quantity and higher quality foods.

Phase 3: continue to eat less/better and get active in a way you enjoy frequently.

Salutation

I hope the tools and strategies contained in this book help you to achieve your weight loss goals. It is possible. You can do it; you just need the right motivation. You just have to want it bad enough.

Once you find your reasons/motivations, remember them every meal. If you take this journey one meal and one snack at a time, before you know it you will have to start increasing your meal portions to maintain your desired weight.

Thanks

Aaron Iacino Certified Nurse Nutritionist Instructor

Copyright 12/10/2012

Recipes

Pasta Primavera

It's a low carb twist on the original. It's basically spaghetti with veggies. But instead of carby noodles we will use sautéed onions as noodles. It's best to use homemade marinara for this and all dishes requiring marinara. You don't have to be a master chef to pull off a good homemade marinara either. All you have to do is use fresh tomatoes or canned chopped, diced or whole tomatoes, crushed garlic, basil, oregano, olive oil, and onions. First sauté the onions with the olive oil until caramelized. Then, lower the heat and add the tomatoes, and dried seasonings. Low and slow baby. Cook the tomatoes on a low heat for a long time and something magical happens. After about two hours or so bam you have marinara sauce. It's crazy, I know. The slow cooking broke down the identity of the tomatoes making a sauce out of them.

You can add whatever veggies you want into the sauce or serve them on top. I like to add black beans and Salmon right into the sauce as its slow cooking. As far as the garlic goes if you want a strong garlic flavor, then add the crushed and minced garlic in at the very end right before you serve it. The more you cook your garlic the less you will taste it just like with onions.

To make the onion noodles; cut them like you were making onion rings and then cut the ring open. The goal is to make them into noodle shapes. Next sauté them until they are at your desired texture.

When you go to plate, lay the onion noodles down first as you would regular noodles. Then, ladle your marinara sauce on top and enjoy.

Once you try the Pasta Primavera with black beans and Salmon you will see why I like it. It has rich, savory and decadent layers of flavors and it will definitely satisfy you and all levels. You will have sweetness from the slow cooked tomatoes, richness from the good fat in the Salmon, and meatiness from the black beans.

The best thing about this recipe is that you can eat a plate full and not just a fist sized portion. The only calories are from the olive oil, beans, and salmon. There will only be a fist portion of these ingredients on your whole plate depending on the amounts you add to the sauce. If you are making a large pot full I would use one can of black beans a two to three 2X2 squares of Salmon.

Seafood Stir-fry

Here is a dish that tastes like $100.00. It is one my favorites, it is super rich while leaving you feeling light. You will not be hungry in an hour either because there is nothing in here to spike your blood sugar.

Use sautéed onions or celery as noodles

Lobster, crab, salad shrimp

Red, yellow and green peppers

Garlic

Season with Bragg soy sauce

Olive oil

Cut onions or celery into desired noodle shape and sauté in a skillet with seafood, crushed and minced garlic, green, red and yellow bell peppers of your choice. Use Bragg brand soy sauce to taste and cook until desired texture is reached. You will not need to add any salt due to the soy sauce. You can add some nuts for more crunch and texture if you're into that. If you like heat, add some crushed red pepper flakes and black pepper.

Once again, you can eat a large portion of this dish because it will only contain a fist full of calorie containing food in it. The calories will come from the seafood and olive oil.

You will be blown away by the flavor of this dish. The Bragg liquid Amino Soy Sauce will rival the flavoring at your favorite Chinese place.

Left Over Stuffing

Do you have a ton of leftover Thanksgiving food that you are running out of options for preparing it? Here is a simple way to enjoy eating it and to save it from the trash can.

Cut all those dinner rolls up that are starting to get hard into ½ inch by ½ inch squares and place into a large mixing bowl.

Next add up your left over Thanksgiving meat cut into small chunks into the mixing bowl. Turkey works well but ham tastes even better.

Next, add your left over gravy into the mixing bowl.

Sauté some onions add season them with some dry herbs. I like to use red pepper flake, oregano, and basil but that's my taste. Once your onions are sautéed add them to the mixing bowl oil and all.

I like to crush and mince up about four cloves of garlic and add it to the mix as well.

Last, grate some cheese up and add in to the mix.

Mix all the ingredients thoroughly and dump them into a baking pan. I use a glass baking dish with two inch walls. I also spray a light coating of cooking spray in the pan first.

Level out the mixture in the pan and bake at 375 degrees until it reaches your desired stuffing texture. I like mine firm, not soggy but not too dry either.

Once you try this stuffing you will never make it the other way again. This takes stuffing from a side dish to a main course.

As far as the Fist Diet goes, this is definitely a calorie containing food so you should only eat a fist sized portion. But on the bright side you now have lunch for about two weeks and you didn't have to waste all those leftovers you were getting sick of by now.

Homemade Refried Beans

Choose your favorite type of beans canned or raw. If raw follow the directions on the package or cook in a pressure cooker. If using canned beans make sure you rinse them, heat in a large sauce pan with chicken stock or water. The more liquid you put in them the longer they will have to cook to reach a thick texture. Mash the cooked beans like you were making mashed potatoes.

Season to taste; I like sautéed onions, crushed and minced garlic, dry basil & oregano, salt, pepper, red pepper flake, raw onions, fresh chopped cilantro, and hot sauce.

Feel free to mix up the beans you use. My favorite is black beans or pinto, but I have used every kind I could buy canned at the store. Sometimes I mix several different kinds to change it up.

Add whatever you think would taste good in them. I have put many different kinds of meats in mine. Cook until they reach your desired thickness.

I like to put two to three tablespoons onto a small flour tortilla with a couple pinches of shredded cheese and fold like a taco. At work, I will place the burrito/taco into the toaster and the heat dial maxed out. When it pops up the contents are warm, the tortilla is crisp, and the cheese is melted.

Two of these for a lunch work great for phase 1 or 2 of the Fist Diet. It is nutrient dense due to the protein created by combining the amino acids of the tortilla and beans, and from the complex carbs and fiber of the beans.

Frittatas

Lube up your baking pan. And dump 15 eggs into it and spread yokes evenly. Add all your leftovers into it and season to taste. Bake 350 until firm. Cut into 15 squares. Now you have breakfast for 5-7 days.

This will work for Phase 1 or 2 of the Fist Diet. It is simple fast and nutrient dense. Eggs are one of the best forms of proteins for humans on the planet.

By cutting the frittatas into in amount of eggs you put in the pan it is easy to get an approximate calorie count. Eggs are about 80 calories per egg. Depending on the leftovers you put in the mix, each square will be approximately 100 calories. You can pound two to three of these babies for breakfast for Phase 1 or 2 of the Fist Diet.

You can eat them cold, warm, or hot. You can even bake and cut them like a pizza. It will actually look like a pizza too, especially if you top it with shredded cheese.

Homemade Gazpacho

Blend raw vegetables in your blender, mostly tomatoes, and season to taste. You can eat it cold or pour into a sauce pan heat and serve. I like to drink it in a glass while hot. You can add meat or whatever you want to give it more substance.

If you need a negative or zero calorie snack, this could qualify depending on if you added calorie containing meats or other ingredients. Blending the veggies whole keeps all the fiber and plant matter. The plant matter (cellulose) is loaded with fiber and is really hard for your body to break down. This is really good for burning any calories that might be contained in the veggies.

Warrior's Chow

Cook or steam rice, wild grain or brown is way better than minute white rice. The minute white turns almost immediately into sugar. The brown or wild rice takes a lot longer to break down, is and loaded with complex carbs and fiber. Add cooked and rinsed beans of your choice (I like black beans). Next add cooked and seasoned ground beef to the pan. After you plate it, top the mix with steamed veggies, salsa, and sprouts.

This dish is called Warrior's Chow for two reasons. First, the mix looks like dog chow. That's why we top it and make it look pretty. Remember we eat with our eyes as much as with our tongue. Second, it has enough protein and complex carbs to carry a warrior through a battle.

Here are some other seasoning options: raw cilantro, sautéed onions, hot sauce, avocados, salt, pepper, and lightly cooked fresh garlic.

Apostle's Salad

Here is a salad for all of you out there who are not afraid of flavor. Use raw dark greens mixed with iceberg lettuce, sun-died tomato vinaigrette, artichoke hearts, green olives, feta cheese, avocados, and diced raw tomatoes.

Those of you practicing the Fist Diet can enjoy a regular sized bowl of this delicious dish on Phase 1 or 2. It contains lots of calories from the dressing, Feta cheese, and avocados but if removed from your bowl they should only amount to a fist size.

This salad is so flavorful and creamy it will satisfy the palate of any respectable foodie.

Homemade Hummus

Hummus is so yummy and creamy it is a wonder that it is dairy free. I got tired of paying too much, for too little, for too many chemical ingredients. Making homemade hummus is quick and easy. Plus you can experiment with different flavors and textures to customize it to your palate. We tried many different flavors from chipotle to feta to black bean. What I have found is that I prefer the original flavor the best.

Ingredients:

> 1 16 oz. can of chickpeas or garbanzo beans
>
> ¼cup liquid from can of chickpeas
>
> ¼ cup of lemon juice (depending on taste)
>
> 1 ½ tablespoons tahini
>
> 4 cloves of raw garlic (crushed)
>
> ½ teaspoon salt
>
> 2 tablespoons olive oil
>
> 1 teaspoon of cumin

Drain chickpeas and set aside liquid from can. Combine remaining ingredients in blender or food processor. Add 1/4 cup of liquid from chickpeas. Blend for 3-5 minutes on low until thoroughly mixed and smooth.

Blend and serve with Special K chips or a fist size of prebaked broken up pizza dough pieces.

Cashew Chicken

Do you love cashew chicken at your favorite Asian buffet? Here is a dish that is easy, quick and healthy.

Sautee onions, garlic, bell peppers, chicken, and cashews in a skillet, cut all ingredients into desired size or the same size chunks. Season the mixture with Bragg's liquid amino acid soy sauce, and pepper, no extra salt. The Bragg will give you plenty of salty flavor.

You can inhale a plateful of this stuff if you want to on either phase 1 or 2 of the Fist Diet. The only calories will come from the oil, chicken and cashews. If you picked out all those calorie containing ingredients it would only add up to a fist full.

Beef and Broccoli

Here is another Asian restaurant inspired dish. Sautee thin sliced beef with small pieces of broccoli and season with Bragg's liquid amino acid soy sauce, pepper, garlic and no extra salt the Bragg will give you plenty of salty flavor. If you are a fan of this dish at your local buffet, you will be even happier with this one at home.

Since half of this dish is the beef, it wouldn't qualify for the plateful loophole. If you are on Phase 1 or 2 of the Fist Diet, then this should be consumed in fist sized portions.

Homemade Salsa

If you are a salsa nut, why not start making your own at home? There are endless recipes and 99% of them are easy as making a peanut butter and jelly sandwich.

Diced tomatoes

Lime or lemon juice

Cilantro

Onions

Garlic

Diced hot peppers if desired

Season with salt, pepper, and dry herbs

Cut everything into small pieces, mix and serve, use as a sauce, topping, a main dish with Special K chips or a couple baked and broken flour tortillas.

I like to make mine like Pico De Gallo, meaning that it is chunkier and contains less liquid, however if you want a restaurant style consistency, then use crushed tomatoes instead of diced tomatoes.

This is a negative or zero calorie dish, so you can eat this all day long without adding to your waistline. You would, however, have to eat it with a spoon.

Homemade Guacamole

Guacamole is the cream cheese of the vegetable/fruit world. Avocados are the stars of this dish and are so creamy you will think you are eating dairy.

Avocados (smashed)

Onions

Cilantro

Dices tomatoes

Season with salt, pepper, hot sauce, hot diced peppers

Dice all ingredients, mix and serve with Special K chips, or use as a topping.

This is a negative or zero calorie snack by itself, so you can eat this all day long if you want to. I know the negative calorie gurus will say that Avocados are not negative calorie but I would like to know anyone who ever gained a pound eating avocados. They do contain good HDL fats (that lower cholesterol) but those same fats help to sustain and satisfy you, thus less food cravings and less food ingesting. When we are satisfied with what we eat we are less likely to inhale some trash foods we found in our cupboards for an after dinner snack.

Butternut Squash Mash

Here is one of my favorite new side dishes. The flavor is so new and unique your taste buds will need a minute to process their new stimulus.

Roast halved gutted butternut squash until you can push a fork into them easily. Let cool, scoop out all meat into a mixing bowl. Smash and mix until smooth. Serve like mashed potatoes, season with salt, pepper, and butter. I like to add a hint of habanero sauce to them. The combination of mashed butternut squash and habanero is ground breaking. Of course you could go normal style and season with gravy.

Unfortunately, butternut squash is a little on the carby side, but it is loaded with so much phytonutrients, vitamins, and minerals it is unbelievable. This dish is on the edge of the zero or negative calorie veggie list, but even in fist sized portions this dish will not let your taste buds or nutrient needs down.

Sweet Potato Soup

Here is another out of the box dishes. Using sweet potatoes instead of regular mashed potatoes will take your nutrient levels through the roof. Any veggie that has this intense color is jam packed with vitamins, minerals, and phytonutrients.

Roast peeled sweet potatoes then blend them in a blender with chicken stock and or milk. Pour into a large sauce pan and add sweet potato chunks, season with salt, pepper, crisp bacon pieces.

This soup is not a zero or negative calorie soup due to the calories contained in the sweet potatoes. Eat in fist sized portions for full unique flavor and a ton of nutrients.

Mud Bars

If I have ten contributions to the world of health and eating, this recipe would have to be in the top three. Mud bars help me get out of bed in the morning. I am only addressing those of you out there that have a sweet tooth the size of King Kong's K-9.

They are definitely not zero or negative calorie. But they are nutrient dense. Depending on how big you make your squares, you could eat two to three of these for a meal on Phase 1 or 2 of the Fist Diet.

From the super healthy peanut butter you will get protein, complex carbs, fiber, (HDL) High Density Lipoproteins (These are the good kinds of fats that remove cholesterol from your body). Plus the good fat in the peanut butter will keep you satisfied and sustained. From the organic oats you will get more complex carbs and fiber. From the honey you will get quick energy to help you get going and out of this world flavor. From the mixed chopped bakers nuts you will get more complex carbs, protein and fiber.

Buy the peanut butter with 1-3 ingredients only. Sometimes it's the kind with the oil on the top or in the refrigerated section. I know that's gross and doesn't taste very good but you are not making a PBJ out of it, we are using it as an ingredient. The other peanut butter has a list of twenty ingredients including sugar. We don't want the added sugar or all the chemicals. I know the chemical peanut butters we grew up on will last longer, but these mud bars will not last long in your fridge anyway (trust me).

Honey is usually 100% pure to start with, but it won't hurt to check for other ingredients. I personally don't care for the taste of the honey that is darker and comes from bees in Asia. I must not be used to the nectar from those flowers. Spend the extra money a get the best purest ingredients you can. Your taste buds will thank you.

Baker's nuts: These are finely chopped mixed nuts. There are usually no peanuts in the mix. Baker's nuts are my favorite to add to Mud Bars. I have used minced walnuts in the past as well as various trail mixes. All these variations were good for different reasons. Experiment until you find what suits you. I will give you a friendly warning however. Frozen raisins are harmful to your smile, use caution. If you use a trail mix with raisins or dried cranberries, make sure you store them in the fridge and not in the freezer.

Organic chopped oats; you can use whole or chopped. I like the chopped due to their texture and better adhesive qualities. The oats add nutrients but are mainly so you don't get your fingers sticky when you eat them.

Here is how I prepare them: mix peanut butter, honey and bakers nuts together in a large mixing bowl (peanut butter to honey ratio is 2 parts peanut butter to 1 part honey, I use 2 lbs. of peanut butter and 1 lbs. of honey), line a cake pan with the oats and pour in the mix, even out the Mud Bar mix and top with oats, place in the freezer for 45 minutes, cut into desired shape and size, bag, store in freezer or refrigerator.

This is not a cheap dish, but protein never is. If you cut your Mud Bars into 15 squares they will cost approximately $1.30 a square.

Green Chili Chicken Enchiladas

I call them enchiladas because Mexican lasagna didn't sound as professional. But how you prepare this dish compares more easily to how you make lasagna.

Corn tortillas

Cream of chicken, or celery, or mushroom soup as sauce

Shredded cheese

Diced green chilies

Shredded chicken

Coat your baking dish with a light coating of oil. Lay down a single layer of small corn tortillas and top them with the soup and diced green chili mix. Next add a layer of shredded chicken and then cheese. Continue the layering process until the pan is full or you run out of a layer. Top with the sauce mix and cheese. Bake until the cheese is melted and it is warm in the center.

I like to cut and plate in squares. You could top it with some un-chopped cilantro. If your end product is too dry, don't panic; just top it with your homemade salsa or guacamole. The next time you make it, just use more of the sauce mix.

This is a flavorful satisfying dish that should be enjoyed in fist sized portions.

Buffalo Chicken Pizza

Oh yeah, this is one of the best nontraditional pizza recipes ever. Most buffalo pizzas you get from the chains skimp on the buffalo sauce to please the heataphobics out there. This is not that pizza. Here are the ingredients:

One whole bottle of Frank's wing sauce

Two packets of Pizza dough mix (or make your own)

Three to four cooked and shredded chicken breasts

Your choice of shredded cheese

Crushed and minced fresh garlic

Prepare dough according to the directions and make sure you include the rest time. Spread dough evenly onto a slightly oiled cookie sheet. Pour whole bottle of Buffalo sauce on dough. Spread shredded chicken on top of sauce. If you put the chicken on top of the cheese like normal it will dry out. The sauce will help the chicken not dry out as well and the cheese blanket on top of it, next spread out garlic and cheese. Bake until the crust is golden brown. I like to stick my finger into the center of the pizza to make sure it is cooked throughout.

This should be enjoyed in fist sized portions.

Creamy Tomato Soup

Creamy tomato soup is a flavor explosion. You get all the tomato flavor infused with the richness of a creamy soup. Here are the ingredients I use:

Crushed tomatoes

Milk or heavy cream

Cilantro

Cheese

Cooked and seasoned thin cut steak strips

Cook all together in a large sauce pan and serve.

This dish should be enjoyed in fist sized portions.

Daily Idolatry
The Fist Diet For Believers
A Scriptural approach to weight loss

Scriptural Strength

Philippians 3:17-21 Brethren, be followers together of me, and mark them which walk so as ye have us for an ensample. (For many walk, of whom I have told you often, and now tell you even weeping, that they are the enemies of the cross of Christ: Whose end is destruction, whose God is their belly, and whose glory is in their shame, who mind earthly things.) For our conversation is in heaven; from whence also we look for the Saviour, the Lord Jesus Christ: Who shall change our vile body, that it may be fashioned like unto his glorious body, according to the working whereby he is able even to subdue all things unto himself.

I don't know about you, but I do not want to be an enemy of the cross of Christ. I don't want to serve my own carnal desires (belly) which will lead me to destruction. I can't wait to get out of this vile flesh and receive my new glorified body on the way up to Heaven in the rapture.

Psalms 144:1 Blessed be the LORD my strength, which teacheth my hands to war, and my fingers to fight: 2 My goodness, and my fortress; my high tower, and my deliverer; my shield, and he in whom I trust.

Scriptural Strength

*Galatians 5:19 Now the works of the flesh are manifest, which are these; Adultery, fornication, uncleanness, lasciviousness, 20 **Idolatry**, witchcraft, hatred, variance, emulations, wrath, strife, seditions, heresies, 21 Envyings, murders, drunkenness, revellings, and such like: of the which I tell you before, as I have also told you in time past, **that they which do such things shall not inherit the kingdom of God.***

I don't know about you, but fear is a huge motivator for me. The thought that I might be in trouble with God and miss out on Heaven is one of the greatest reasons I live the way I live. If I take that same fear and apply it to misusing food, I will not replace God with a doughnut or a bag of chips. Sounds crazy right? But a lot of us misuse food for the comfort and anxiety reductions we should be seeking in God.

Definition of Idolatry

The worship of idols; the worship of images that are not God.[Wordnet]

The worship of idols, images, or anything which is not God; the worship of false gods.[Websters]

Excessive attachment or veneration for anything; respect or love which borders on adoration.[Websters].

Idolatry, in Christian theology, is "the worship of a created object" rather than the true God. The term "idol" often refers to conceptual constructs such as fame, money, nationality, ethnicity, and the ritual of attachment related to these is considered idolatry. Because a knowledge of God is supposed to transcend the conceptual, residing instead within people's emotional understanding, the theological concept of idolatry is related to the psychological concept of attachment.

Source - Webster's Dictionary

If I put anything in the place of God it is defined as idolatry. If I use food as my comforter when God sent His Spirit to be my comforter, then am I committing idolatry? If I turn to food when I am overwhelmed instead of turning to God, then did I make food my god?

Scriptural Strength

*Colossians 5 Mortify therefore your members which are upon the earth; fornication, uncleanness, **inordinate affection**, evil concupiscence, and covetousness, **which is idolatry**: 6 For which things' sake the wrath of God* *cometh on the children of disobedience: 7 In the which ye also walked some time, when ye lived in them.*

John 14:10-18 Believe me that I am in the Father, and the Father in me: or else believe me for the very works' sake. Verily, verily, I say unto you, He that believeth on me, the works that I do shall he do also; ***and greater works than these shall he do;*** *because I go unto my Father. And whatsoever ye shall ask in my name, that will I do, that the Father may be glorified in the Son. If ye shall ask any thing in my name, I will do it. If ye love me, keep my commandments.* ***And I will pray the Father, and he shall give you another Comforter, that he may abide with you for ever;*** *Even the Spirit of truth; whom the world cannot receive, because it seeth him not, neither knoweth him: but ye know him; for he dwelleth with you, and shall be in you. I will not leave you comfortless: I will come to you.*

*John 14:26-****27 But the Comforter, which is the Holy Ghost, whom the Father will send in my name, he shall teach you all things,*** *and bring all things to your remembrance, whatsoever I have said unto you.* ***Peace I leave with you, my peace I give unto you****: not as the world giveth, give I unto you. Let not your heart be troubled, neither let it be afraid.*

If I am replacing the comfort I should be getting from God with "comfort food", then am I opening myself up for the wrath of God?

Galatians 6:7 Be not deceived; God is not mocked: for whatsoever a man soweth, that shall he also reap. ***8 For he that soweth to his flesh shall of the flesh reap corruption****; but he that soweth to the Spirit shall of the Spirit reap life everlasting.*

If I allow my flesh to rule me, it will want to eat bad food all the time and in huge portions. If I sow this lifestyle I will reap a huge weight gain. My flesh does not care if I am fat. It just wants to party. It knows that it will not go to Heaven or hell.

1 Corinthians 15:50 Now this I say, brethren, ***that flesh and blood cannot inherit the kingdom of God****; neither doth corruption inherit incorruption.*

*Hebrews 13: 7-9 Remember them which have the rule over you, who have spoken unto you the word of God: whose faith follow, considering the end of their conversation. Jesus Christ the same yesterday, and to day, and for ever. Be not carried about with divers and strange doctrines. **For it is a good thing that the heart be established with grace; not with meats, which have not profited them that have been occupied therein.***

If the purpose of our life is to serve our stomach we'll receive no profit. If our Heart (mind) is occupied with Jesus, than he will establish us.

Motivation

Weak or no motivation = no change in body

What is your motivation?

Looking for your missing rib?

Want to make a beautiful Temple for God's Spirit?

Do you want more time to serve God?

Do you want to enjoy the life God gave you?

Market Motivation

*Genesis 2:18-25 **And the LORD God said, It is not good that the man should be alone;** I will make him an help meet for him. And out of the ground the LORD God formed every beast of the field, and every fowl of the air; and brought them unto Adam to see what he would call them: and whatsoever Adam called every living creature, that was the name thereof. And Adam gave names to all cattle, and to the fowl of the air, and to every beast of the field; but for Adam there was not found an help meet for him. And the LORD God caused a deep sleep to fall upon Adam, and he slept: and he took one of his ribs, and closed up the flesh instead thereof; And the rib, which the LORD God had taken from man, made he a woman, and* brought her unto the man. And Adam said, This is now bone of my bones, and flesh of my flesh: she shall be called Woman, because she was taken out of Man. Therefore shall a man leave his father and his mother, and shall cleave unto his wife: and they shall be one flesh. And they were both naked, the man and his wife, and were not ashamed.

Genesis 1: 28-29 **And God blessed them, and God said unto them, Be fruitful, and multiply, and replenish the earth**, *and subdue it: and have dominion over the fish of the sea, and over the fowl of the air, and over every living thing that moveth upon the earth. 29And God said, Behold, I have given you every herb bearing seed, which is upon the face of all the earth, and every tree, in the which is the fruit of a tree yielding seed; to you it shall be for meat.*

Genesis 9:1 And God blessed Noah and his sons, and said unto them, **Be fruitful, and multiply,** *and replenish the earth.*

It is Godly to be seeking your other half. God commanded us to be fruitful and multiply. Getting to your ideal weight/shape will give you the confidence need to get out there and find your missing rib/side.

Glorify God Motivation

1 Corinthians 16:19 **What? know ye not that your body is the temple of the Holy Ghost which is in you,** *which ye have of God, and ye are not your own? 20 For ye are bought with a price:* **therefore glorify God in your body,** *and in your spirit, which are God's.*

Acts 2:36- 41 Now when they heard this, they were pricked in their heart, and said unto Peter and to the rest of the apostles, Men and brethren, what shall we do? **Then Peter said unto them, Repent, and be baptized every one of you in the name of Jesus Christ for the remission of sins, and ye shall receive the gift of the Holy Ghost. For the promise is unto you, and to your children, and to all that are afar off, even as many as the Lord our God shall call.** *And with many other words did he testify and exhort, saying, Save yourselves from this untoward generation. Then they* *that gladly received his word were baptized: and the same day there were added unto them about three thousand souls.*

When you become filled with the Spirit of God, you are in fact a temple of the Holy Ghost. If we want to glorify God in our bodies we should not permit the flesh to control our outward image. Whatever is on the inside of us, will show on the outside of us. If I am a biker in heart, I will look like a biker on the outside.

If we are permitting God to control us with His Word, and are battling our flesh daily to live holy on the inside, we will also look holy on the outside. If we are battling and overcoming our flesh to live holy we can use that same skill to battle our flesh at the dinner table.

Scriptural Strength

*John 17:1 These words spake Jesus, and lifted up his eyes to heaven, and said, Father, the hour is come; glorify thy Son, that thy Son also may glorify thee: 2 **As thou hast given him power over all flesh**, that he should give eternal life to as many as thou hast given him.*

*Phil 4:12 I know both how to be abased, and I know how to abound: every where and in all things I am instructed both to be full and to be hungry, both to abound and to suffer need. 13 **I can do all things through Christ which strengtheneth me.***

We can accomplish all things through the strength of our Lord Jesus, even weight loss. If you have followed His plan of salvation, then He already gave you the power to follow Him instead of your flesh. If you followed His plan of salvation, then you already turned on your flesh and turned to Him. It's time to realize the power we have through Christ. We can overcome eating too much if we trust in God and have faith in the power of His might over our flesh.

When you've decided to turn on yourself and follow Christ, you had to deny yourself. If you have been saved a little while, then you are becoming a master of not doing what your flesh wants you to do.

Why then do we deny our flesh when it wants to cuss or lust, but we do not deny it when it wants to kill us with the spoon?

The Main Enemy

Proverbs 13:25 The righteous eateth to the satisfying of his soul: but the belly of the wicked shall want.

Flesh is our main enemy. Even if we gave it to eat what it wants, when it wants it, the amount it craves; It still would not be satisfied.

Matthew 15:17 Do not ye yet understand, that whatsoever entereth in at the mouth goeth into the belly, and is cast out into the draught?

To allow our flesh to idolize food that turns into feces, is a waste of our time, and will only lead to depression.

1 Corinthians 6:12-13 All things are lawful unto me, but all things are not expedient: all things are lawful for me, but I will not be brought under the power of any. Meats for the belly, and the belly for meats: but God shall destroy both it and them. Now the body is not for fornication, but for the Lord; and the Lord for the body.

We must take the same stance here as Brother Paul. We cannot allow ourselves to be brought under the power of food. We must instead submit ourselves to the authority of God's Word through the anointed vessels He gave us. Both our bodies and all the food in the world is eventually going to be destroyed, but our soul will live forever. We must take heed to the spiritual matters in life over our flesh if we want to spend eternity in Heaven.

Romans 16:17-18 Now I beseech you, brethren, mark them which cause divisions and offences contrary to the doctrine which ye have learned; and avoid them. For they that are such serve not our Lord Jesus Christ, but their own belly; and by good words and fair speeches deceive the hearts of the simple.

Notice how the Apostle Paul uses the term "belly" to describe serving our own carnal desires.

Romans 8:1-16 **There is therefore now no condemnation to them which are in Christ Jesus, who walk not after the flesh, but after the Spirit.** *For the law of the Spirit of life in Christ Jesus hath made me free from the law of sin and death. For what the law could not do, in that it was weak through the flesh, God sending his own Son in the likeness of sinful flesh, and for sin, condemned sin in the flesh: That the righteousness of the law might be fulfilled in us, who walk not after the flesh, but after the Spirit. For they that are after the flesh do mind the things of the flesh; but they that are after the Spirit the things of the Spirit.* **For to be carnally minded is death;** *but to be spiritually minded is life and peace.* **Because the carnal mind is enmity against God:** *for it is not subject to the law of God, neither indeed can be. So then they that are in the flesh cannot please God. But ye are not in the flesh, but in the Spirit, if so be that the Spirit of God dwell in you. Now if any man have not the Spirit of Christ, he is none of his. And if Christ be in you, the body is dead because of sin; but the Spirit is life because of righteousness. But if the Spirit of him that raised up Jesus from the dead dwell in you, he that raised up Christ from the dead shall also quicken your mortal bodies by his Spirit that dwelleth in you. Therefore, brethren, we are debtors, not to the flesh, to live after the flesh.* **For if ye live after the flesh, ye shall die: but if ye through the Spirit do mortify the deeds of the body, ye shall live.** *For as many as are led by the Spirit of God, they are the sons of God. For ye have not received the spirit of bondage again to fear; but ye have received the Spirit of adoption, whereby we cry, Abba, Father. The Spirit itself beareth witness with our spirit, that we are the children of God:*

If we allow our flesh to run wild every meal time and snack time it will eventually kill us. Our unredeemed human nature cannot do the right thing. The flesh is an enemy of God and does not want you to glorify God with your body. The flesh wants you to glorify it.

Romans 13:11 And that, knowing the time, that now it is high time to awake out of sleep: for now is our salvation nearer than when we believed. The night is far spent, the day is at hand: let us therefore cast off the works of darkness, and let us put on the armour of light. Let us walk honestly, as in the day; not in rioting and drunkenness, not in chambering and wantonness, not in strife and envying. But put ye on the Lord Jesus Christ, **and make not provision for the flesh, to fulfil the lusts thereof.**

If you give your flesh an inch it will take a mile. If we make provisions for it to have its way at meal time, it will not stop and before we know it we are overweight.

Ephesians 2:1 And you hath he quickened, who were dead in trespasses and sins; 2 Wherein in time past ye walked according to the course of this world, according to the prince of the power of the air, the spirit that now worketh in the children of disobedience: 3 **Among whom also we all had our conversation in times past in the lusts of our flesh, fulfilling the desires of the flesh and of the mind;** *and were by nature the children of wrath, even as others.*

Romans 6:11-16 Likewise reckon ye also yourselves to be dead indeed unto sin, but alive unto God through Jesus Christ our Lord. Let not sin therefore reign in your mortal body, **that ye should obey it in the lusts thereof.** *Neither yield ye your members as instruments of unrighteousness unto sin: but yield yourselves unto God, as those that are alive from the dead, and your members as instruments of righteousness unto God. For sin shall not have dominion over you: for ye are not under the law, but under grace. What then? shall we sin, because we are not under the law, but under grace? God forbid.* **Know ye not, that to whom ye yield yourselves servants to obey, his servants ye are to whom ye obey;** *whether of sin unto death, or of obedience unto righteousness?*

Before we were saved we did whatever our flesh wanted us to do. We were slaves to our carnal human desires. Now that we are made alive and have been pardoned for all of our sins, why not walk in that newness of life? We have the power over our flesh now. The old excuse of "I can't help it" will not get us into the Kingdom of God. Why do we still use that excuse at meal time?

The Other Enemy

Matthew 4:1-4 Then was Jesus led up of the Spirit into the wilderness to be tempted of the devil. 2 And when he had fasted forty days and forty nights, he was afterward an hungered. 3 And when the tempter came to him, he said, If thou be the Son of God, command that these stones be made bread. 4 But he answered and said, It is written, **Man shall not live by bread alone, but by every word that proceedeth out of the mouth of God.**

Isn't funny how the devil is using food to try to get Jesus to sin? Why would the devil change his strategy, it worked with Adam and Eve to get all of mankind to fall. Don't put it past your flesh to use food to get you to fall. The devil and the flesh work together. They know that food is a weak point for humanity. It is the small foxes that destroy the vine. Don't let your flesh use your bodies' weakness against you. Fight the flesh and push the plate away

Genesis 3:4 And the serpent said unto the woman, **Ye shall not surely die***: 5 For God doth know that in the day ye eat thereof, then your eyes shall be opened, and ye shall be as gods, knowing good and evil. 6 And when the woman saw that the tree was good for food, and that it was pleasant to the eyes, and a tree to be desired to make one wise, she took of the fruit thereof, and did eat, and gave also unto her husband with her; and he did eat.*

Scriptural Strength

Psalms 91:15 He shall call upon me, and I will answer him: I will be with him in trouble; I will deliver him, and honour him. 16 With long life will I satisfy him, and show him my salvation.

In our relationship with God comes our satisfaction, real true satisfaction. Food is only temporarily satisfying and it only satisfies the flesh. Our walk with God is satisfying right down to the depth of our very souls. There is nothing more satisfying than being right with the almighty creator. God will be there with us when we are weak, He will deliver us from trouble. If you are trying to deny your flesh at meal time and are struggling, He can help.

Isa 58:11 And the LORD shall guide thee continually, and satisfy thy soul in drought, and make fat thy bones: and thou shalt be like a watered garden, and like a spring of water, whose waters fail not.

*Exodus 16:2 And the whole congregation of the children of Israel murmured against Moses and Aaron in the wilderness: 3 And the children of Israel said unto them, Would to God we had died by the hand of the LORD in the land of Egypt, **when we sat by the flesh pots, and when we did eat bread to the full**; for ye have brought us forth into this wilderness, to kill this whole assembly with hunger.*

No Hebrew entered into the promise land over the age of forty except for Caleb and Joshua. All the rest of the people God refused entry. One of the biggest reasons for God's rejection of them was for their complaining. Guess what they were complaining about? You guessed it, food. They wanted to be full. Eating to get full at mealtime will lead to weight gain. It's only our flesh that craves that full feeling. Our body does not need a full tank to run off. In fact God designed our bodies to run off an empty tank. God required fasting throughout the Bible and still calls for it today. Recent studies have shown that the energy we get from using our fat storages causes an increase in energy and mental acuity.

Isaiah 58:1-14 Cry aloud, spare not, lift up thy voice like a trumpet, and show my people their transgression, and the house of Jacob their sins. Yet they seek me daily, and delight to know my ways, as a nation that did righteousness, and forsook not the ordinance of their God: they ask of me the ordinances of justice; they take delight in approaching to God. Wherefore have we fasted, say they, and thou seest not? wherefore have we afflicted our soul, and thou takest no knowledge? Behold, in the day of your fast ye find pleasure, and exact all your labours. Behold, ye fast for strife and debate, and to smite with the fist of wickedness: ye shall not fast as ye do this day, to make your voice to be heard on high. Is it such a fast that I have chosen? a day for a man to afflict his soul? is it to bow down his head as a bulrush, and to spread sackcloth and ashes under him? wilt thou call this a fast, and an acceptable day to the LORD? **Is not this the fast that I have chosen? to loose the bands of wickedness, to undo the heavy burdens, and to let the oppressed go free, and that ye break every yoke?** Is it not to deal thy bread to the hungry, and that thou bring the poor that are cast out to thy house? when thou seest the naked, that thou cover him; and that thou hide not thyself from thine own flesh? **Then shall thy light break forth as the morning, and thine health shall spring forth speedily: and thy righteousness shall go before thee; the glory of the LORD shall be thy rereward. Then shalt thou call, and the LORD shall answer; thou shalt cry, and he shall say, Here I am. If thou take away from the midst of thee the yoke, the putting forth of the finger, and speaking vanity; And if thou draw out thy soul to the hungry, and satisfy the afflicted soul; then shall thy light rise in obscurity, and thy darkness be as the noonday: And the LORD shall guide thee continually, and satisfy thy soul in drought, and make fat thy bones: and thou shalt be like a watered garden, and like a spring of water, whose waters fail not.** And they that shall be of thee shall build the old waste places: thou shalt raise up the foundations of many generations; and thou shalt be called, The repairer of the breach, The restorer of paths to dwell in. If thou turn away thy foot from the sabbath, from doing thy pleasure on my holy day; and call the sabbath a delight, the holy of the LORD, honourable; and shalt honour him, not doing thine own ways, nor finding thine own pleasure, nor speaking thine own words: Then shalt thou delight thyself in the LORD; and I will cause thee to ride upon the high places of the earth, and feed thee with the heritage of Jacob thy father: for the mouth of the LORD hath spoken it.

Matthew 17:14-21 And when they were come to the multitude, there came to him a certain man, kneeling down to him, and saying, 15Lord, have mercy on my son: for he is lunatic, and sore vexed: for ofttimes he falleth into the fire, and oft into the water. 16And I brought him to thy *disciples, and they could not cure him. 17Then Jesus answered and said, O faithless and perverse generation, how long shall I be with you? how long shall I suffer you? bring him hither to me. 18And Jesus rebuked the devil; and he departed out of him: and the child was cured from that very hour. 19Then came the disciples to Jesus apart, and said, Why could not we cast him out? 20And Jesus said unto them, Because of your unbelief: for verily I say unto you, If ye have faith as a grain of mustard seed, ye shall say unto this mountain, Remove hence to yonder place; and it shall remove; and nothing shall be impossible unto you. **21Howbeit this kind goeth not out but by prayer and fasting.***

Fist Psych

Food is not an escape from reality

If our life sucks we need to pin point why it sucks and work towards fixing it

If it is beyond repair or if it is going to take several years to get our lives to a point of some comfort then we need find healthy escapes

Prayer, serving God, vacations, hobbies etc...

Scriptural Strength

Psalms 18:2 The LORD is my rock, and my fortress, and my deliverer; my God, my strength, in whom I will trust; my buckler, and the horn of my salvation, and my high tower.

Psalms 61:1 Hear my cry, O God; attend unto my prayer. 2 From the end of the earth will I cry unto thee, when my heart is overwhelmed: lead me to the rock that is higher than I. 3 For thou hast been a shelter for me, and a strong tower from the enemy. 4 I will abide in thy tabernacle for ever: I will trust in the covert of thy wings. Selah

Fist Psych

Food is not entertainment

You do not have to eat while your watch TV or when you are on the computer

You should not eat to cure boredom

Scriptural Strength

*Hebrews 11:6 **But without faith it is impossible to please him**: for he that cometh to God must believe that he is, and that he is a rewarder of them that diligently seek him.*

We could change our focus from pleasing ourselves with food to pleasing God with faith.

*Matthew 8:5 And when Jesus was entered into Capernaum, there came unto him a centurion, beseeching him, 6And saying, Lord, my servant lieth at home sick of the palsy, grievously tormented. 7And Jesus saith unto him, **I will come and heal him.***

*Luke 4: 18 The Spirit of the Lord is upon me, because he hath anointed me to preach the gospel to the poor; **he hath sent me to heal the brokenhearted**, to preach deliverance to the captives, and recovering of sight to the blind, to set at liberty them that are bruised, 19To preach the acceptable year of the Lord.*

*Deuteronomy 32:39 See now that I, even I, am he, and there is no god with me: I kill, and I make alive; I wound, and **I heal**: neither is there any that can deliver out of my hand. 40 For I lift up my hand to heaven, and say, I live for ever.*

1 Sam 2:6-10 The LORD killeth, and maketh alive: he bringeth down to the grave, and bringeth up. The LORD maketh poor, and maketh rich: he

bringeth low, and lifteth up. He raiseth up the poor out of the dust, and lifteth up the beggar from the dunghill, to set them among princes, and to make them inherit the throne of glory: for the pillars of the earth are the LORD'S, and he hath set the world upon them. He will keep the feet of his saints, and the wicked shall be silent in darkness; for by strength shall no man prevail. The adversaries of the LORD shall be broken to pieces; out of heaven shall he thunder upon them: the LORD shall judge the ends of the earth; and he shall give strength unto his king, and exalt the horn of his anointed.

It is true that the nutrients in real foods we eat can heal our bodies. But who made every fruit bearing plant? It is God that ultimately heals us.

*Genesis 1:1-31 In the beginning God created the heaven and the earth. And the earth was without form, and void; and darkness was upon the face of the deep. And the Spirit of God moved upon the face of the waters. And God said, Let there be light: and there was light. And God saw the light, that it was good: and God divided the light from the darkness. And God called the light Day, and the darkness he called Night. And the evening and the morning were the first day. And God said, Let there be a firmament in the midst of the waters, and let it divide the waters from the waters. And God made the firmament, and divided the waters which were under the firmament from the waters which were above the firmament: and it was so. And God called the firmament Heaven. And the evening and the morning were the second day. And God said, Let the waters under the heaven be gathered together unto one place, and let the dry land appear: and it was so. And God called the dry land Earth; and the gathering together of the waters called he Seas: and God saw that it was good. **And God said, Let the earth bring forth grass, the herb yielding seed, and the fruit tree yielding fruit after his kind, whose seed is in itself, upon the earth: and it was so. And the earth brought forth grass, and herb yielding seed after his kind, and the tree yielding fruit, whose seed was in itself, after his kind: and God saw that it was good.** And the evening and the morning were the third day. And God said, Let there be lights in the firmament of the heaven to divide the day from the night; and let* them be for signs, and for seasons, and for days, and years: And let them be for lights in the firmament of the heaven to give light upon the earth: and it was so. And God made two great lights; the greater light to rule the day, and the lesser light to rule the night: he made the stars also. And God set them in the firmament of the heaven to give light upon the earth, And to rule over the day and over the night, and to divide the light from the darkness: and God saw that it was good. And the evening and the morning were the fourth day. And God said, Let the waters bring forth abundantly the moving creature that hath life, and fowl that may fly above the earth in the open firmament of heaven. And God created great whales, and every living creature that moveth, which the waters brought forth abundantly, after their kind, and every winged fowl after his kind: and God saw that it was good. And God blessed them, saying, Be fruitful, and multiply, and fill the waters in the seas, and let fowl multiply in the earth. And the evening and the morning were the fifth day. And God said, Let the earth bring forth the living creature after his kind, cattle, and creeping thing, and beast of the earth after his kind: and it was so. And God made the beast of the earth after his kind, and cattle after their kind, and every thing that creepeth upon the earth after his kind: and God saw that it was good. And God said, Let us make man in our image, after our likeness: and let them have dominion over the fish of the sea, and over the fowl of the air, and over the cattle, and over all the earth, and over every creeping thing that creepeth upon the earth. So God created man in his own image, in the image of God created he him; male and female created he them. And God blessed them, and God said unto them, Be fruitful, and multiply, and replenish the earth, and subdue it: and have dominion over the fish of the sea, and over the fowl of the air, and over every living thing that moveth upon the earth. **And God said, Behold, I have given you every herb bearing seed, which is upon the face of all the earth, and every tree, in the which is the fruit of a tree yielding seed; to you it shall be for meat. And to every beast of the earth, and to every fowl of the air, and to every thing that creepeth upon the earth, wherein there is life, I have given every green herb for meat: and it was so. And God saw every thing** *that he had made, and, behold, it was very good.* And the evening and the morning were the sixth day.

*John 15:1-8 I am the true vine, and my Father is the husbandman. Every branch in me that beareth not fruit he taketh away: and every branch that beareth fruit, he purgeth it, that it may bring forth more fruit. **Now ye are clean through the word which I have spoken unto you.** Abide in me, and I in you. As the branch cannot bear fruit of itself, except it abide in the vine; no more can ye, except ye abide in me. I am the vine, ye are the branches: He that abideth in me, and I in him, the same bringeth forth much fruit: for without me ye can do nothing. If a man abide not in me, he is cast forth as a branch, and is withered; and men gather them, and cast them into the fire, and they are burned. If ye abide in me, and my words abide in you, ye shall ask what ye will, and it shall be done unto you. Herein is my Father glorified, that ye bear much fruit; so shall ye be my disciples.*

There is nothing wrong with undergoing a physical cleansing every now and then. The safe natural products on the market can help your body get rid of all the pollutants from the trash at the food chains. But if it is a deep soul cleaning you are after, then hearing the true unadulterated Word of God is the best cleaner out there.

*Matthew 11:28 Come unto me, all ye that labour and are heavy laden, and **I will give you rest**. 29 Take my yoke upon you, and learn of me; for I am meek and lowly in heart: **and ye shall find rest unto your souls.** 30 For my yoke is easy, and my burden is light.*

There is no better rest when after you eat a huge meal and lay down for a nap right? Actually there is. The rest from being right with God is like no other, the peace that comes from being sure that you are in line with the Word of God, the freedom of the fear of death because you have faith in His Word. This is true rest. This kind of rest/peace triumphs over any money problem or relationship issue, this rest/peace gets the victory over any work problem you might be facing.

James 1:17 Every good gift and every perfect gift is from above, and cometh down from the Father of lights, with whom is no variableness, neither shadow of turning.

It is steeped in every culture to use food as a reward. If we are seeking rewards there is none greater than the gifts that come from God: repentance, forgiveness, and being filled with His Spirit.

*1 Corinthians 10:13 **There hath no temptation taken you but such as is common to man**: but God is faithful, who will not suffer you to be tempted above that ye are able; but will with the temptation also make a way to escape, that ye may be able to bear it. 14 Wherefore, my dearly beloved, flee from idolatry.*

The temptation to overeat and to eat trash food universal and sadly it is also culturally OK to pig out. When you start losing ten pounds and then another ten pounds everyone you know will act like your doctor and start to give you medical advice. They will worry about your health and tell you to lose weight a different way. All these people will be overweight themselves. On the flip side when you were gaining the weight you rarely if ever got a concerning comment from the same people.

Just know that when you are tempted to follow your carnal desires and eat too much, that everyone else is going through the same thing. Take comfort in knowing that through God you can overcome the flesh and tell it "NO" and refuse to overeat.

Married Folks

Hebrews 13:4 Marriage is honourable in all, and the bed undefiled:

1 Corinthians 7: 3 Let the husband render unto the wife due benevolence: and likewise also the wife unto the husband. 4 The wife hath not power of her own body, but the husband: and likewise also the husband hath not power of his own body, but the wife. 5 Defraud ye not one the other, except it be with consent for a time, that ye may give yourselves to fasting and prayer; and come together again, that Satan tempt you not for your incontinency.

*Ephesians 5:25 Husbands, love your wives, even as Christ also loved the church, and gave himself for it; 26 That he might sanctify and cleanse it with the washing of water by the word, 27 That he might present it to himself a glorious church, not having spot, or wrinkle, or any such thing; but that it should be holy and without blemish. 28 **So ought men to love their wives as their own bodies**. He that loveth his wife loveth himself. 29 For no man ever yet hated his own flesh; but nourisheth and cherisheth it, even as the Lord the church: 30 For we are members of his body, of his flesh, and of his bones.*

To truly care for our wives is to care for ourselves. What good are we as husbands to our wives if we are sick all the time or dead. Our overeating and eating trash foods is the main cause for our sicknesses. I know it is easy to blame our wives for our being overweight because in some homes the wife does the majority of the cooking. If we blame her for our excess fat then we are no better then Adam. Eve was deceived and ate the fruit and gave it to her husband. Adam did not have to eat it. He knew better. He could have chosen his relationship with God over his relationship with Eve and sparred all of humanity a sinful nature. We must not follow his lead. If we are being handed too much food that has too many calories, we can still chose not to eat it all. Let us just eat a fist sized portion and watch the pounds fall off.

When we decide to deny our flesh's desire to eat trash and to overeat, we will inspire our significant other. When we start dropping the disease causing fat pounds our spouse will take notice. When meal after meal they see us eating better foods and smaller quantities, it will affect them. We can influence others when we first change ourselves.

When you first got saved and stopped sinning did you notice the affect it had on others? The same transmission affect will happen when you start denying your flesh at meal and snack time.

I am speaking from personal experience. I never told my wife that she should lose weight. I definitely do not recommend anyone ever telling their wife that. I did however start dropping pounds myself and she just jumped on board. I never asked her to, but our bond was tight and I took the lead.

Worst case scenario we have to do what Saint Peter told us to do in Acts 2:40. That is to save ourselves. God gave us all free will and if your spouse refuses to act upon the conviction you have been transmitting, then it should not stop you from getting healthy yourself.

Bacon vs. the Bible

It is OK to eat your favorite meats. Just do it fist sized

*1 Timothy 4:1 Now the Spirit speaketh expressly, that in the latter times some shall depart from the faith, **giving heed to seducing spirits, and doctrines of devils; 2 Speaking lies in hypocrisy;** having their conscience seared with a hot iron; 3 Forbidding to marry, **and commanding to abstain from meats,** which God hath created to be received with thanksgiving of them which believe and know the truth. 4 For every creature of God is good, and nothing to be refused, if it be received with thanksgiving: 5 For it is sanctified by the word of God and prayer.*

*Acts 11:7 And I heard a voice saying unto me, Arise, Peter; slay and eat. 8 But I said, Not so, Lord: for nothing common or unclean hath at any time entered into my mouth. 9 But the voice answered me again from heaven, **What God hath cleansed, that call not thou common.***

These Scriptures are very transparent and should clear up any questions if it is a sin to eat meat. All we have to do to enjoy our bacon is thank God for it.

Daniel 1:1-12 In the third year of the reign of Jehoiakim king of Judah came Nebuchadnezzar king of Babylon unto Jerusalem, and besieged it. And the Lord gave Jehoiakim king of Judah into his hand, with part of the vessels of the house of God: which he carried into the land of Shinar to the *house of his god; and he brought the vessels into the treasure house of his god. And the king spake unto Ashpenaz the master of his eunuchs, that he should bring certain of the children of Israel, and of the king's seed, and of the princes; Children in whom was no blemish, but well favoured, and skilful in all wisdom, and cunning in knowledge, and understanding science, and such as had ability in them to stand in the king's palace, and whom they might teach the learning and the tongue of the Chaldeans. And the king appointed them a daily provision of the king's meat, and of the wine which he drank: so nourishing them three years, that at the end thereof they might stand before the king. Now among these were of the children of Judah, Daniel, Hananiah, Mishael, and Azariah: Unto whom the prince of the eunuchs gave names: for he gave unto Daniel the name of Belteshazzar; and to Hananiah, of Shadrach; and to Mishael, of Meshach; and to Azariah, of Abednego. **But Daniel purposed in his heart that he would not defile himself with the portion of the king's meat, nor with the wine which he drank:** therefore he requested of the prince of the eunuchs that he might not defile himself. Now God had brought Daniel into favour and tender love with the prince of the eunuchs. And the prince of the eunuchs said unto Daniel, I fear my lord the king, who hath appointed your meat and your drink: for why should he see your faces worse liking than the children which are of your sort? then shall ye make me endanger my head to the king. Then said Daniel to Melzar, whom the prince of the eunuchs had set over Daniel, Hananiah, Mishael, and Azariah, Prove thy servants, **I beseech thee, ten days; and let them give us pulse to eat, and water to drink.** Then let our countenances be looked upon before thee, and the countenance of the children that eat of the portion of the king's meat: and as thou seest, deal with thy servants. So he consented to them in this matter, and proved them ten days. **And at the end of ten days their countenances appeared fairer and fatter in flesh than all the children which did eat the portion of the king's meat.** Thus Melzar took away the portion of their meat, and the wine that they should drink; and gave them pulse. **As for these four children, God gave them knowledge and skill in all learning and wisdom: and Daniel had understanding in all visions and dreams.** Now at the end of the days that* *the king had said he should bring them in, then the prince of the eunuchs brought them in before Nebuchadnezzar. And the king communed with them; and among them all was found none like Daniel, Hananiah, Mishael, and Azariah: therefore stood they before the king. And in all matters of wisdom and understanding, that the king inquired of them, he found them ten times better than all the magicians and astrologers that were in all his realm. And Daniel continued even unto the first year of king Cyrus.*

These Scriptures are commonly misused to advocate for vegetarianism. What is a sin in these Scriptures is to eat meat that has been sacrificed to false gods. Daniel knew the Scriptures and knew this was against God's expressed will. Daniel refused to eat the meat and get God angry with him. Instead he ate vegetables and had faith in God. His willing obedience and faith paid off, God rewarded him with a healthier body and a sharper mind then those who defiled themselves.

Nothing good comes without sacrifice. But what are we really sacrificing by controlling our portions, skipping the doughnuts in the break room, and the bag of chips at the gas station. Sure we are missing out on pleasing our flesh for a few minutes, but we are also gaining energy, health, self-esteem, confidence, eradicating diseases, and we are glorifying God in our bodies.

Proverbs 23:19-21 Hear thou, my son, and be wise, and guide thine heart in the way. Be not among winebibbers; among riotous eaters of flesh: For the drunkard and the glutton shall come to poverty: and drowsiness shall clothe a man with rags.

Here in Proverbs, King Solomon is telling us not to even hang out with those overeating, he also states that those who do overeat will come to poverty. I can understand what he is saying from personal experience. I would have had a lot more money in my pockets if I was not giving it to the trash chains and vending machines. When I was obese, I had a lot less energy and a lot more pain, as a result I spent more time on the bed and couch and was a lot less productive at work.

Scriptural Strength

John 4:30 Then they went out of the city, and came unto him. 31In the mean while his disciples prayed him, saying, Master, eat. 32 But he said unto them, **I have meat to eat that ye know not of.** *33 Therefore said the disciples one to another, Hath any man brought him ought to eat? 34 Jesus saith unto them,* **My meat is to do the will of him that sent me, and to finish his work. 35 Say not ye, There are yet four months, and then cometh harvest? behold, I say unto you, Lift up your eyes, and look on the fields; for they are white already to harvest. 36 And he that reapeth receiveth wages, and gathereth fruit unto life eternal: that both he that soweth and he that reapeth may rejoice together. 37 And herein is that saying true, One soweth, and another reapeth. 38 I sent you to reap that whereon ye bestowed no labour: other men laboured, and ye are entered into their labours.**

Once we realize that the source of our strength is God and not food, we can start to take food off the throne we put it on. Food is not god, food cannot keep us alive, food is only a tool.

John 6:24 When the people therefore saw that Jesus was not there, neither his disciples, they also took shipping, and came to Capernaum, seeking for Jesus. 25And when they had found him on the other side of the sea, they said unto him, Rabbi, when camest thou hither? 26Jesus answered them and said, **Verily, verily, I say unto you, Ye seek me, not because ye saw the miracles, but because ye did eat of the loaves, and were filled. 27Labour not for the meat which perisheth, but for that meat which endureth unto everlasting life, which the Son of man shall give unto you: for him hath God the Father sealed.**

Jesus told us that we should desire His Word that will give us everlasting life, instead of focusing on food that rots.

Hebrews 12:14 Follow peace with all men, and holiness, without which no man shall see the Lord: 15Looking diligently lest any man fail of the grace of God; lest any root of bitterness springing up trouble you, and thereby *many be defiled; 16Lest there be any fornicator, or profane person, **as Esau, who for one morsel of meat sold his birthright**. 17For ye know how that afterward, when he would have inherited the blessing, he was rejected: for he found no place of repentance, though he sought it carefully with tears.*

Esau exchanged God's blessing for a temporary feeling. He will no doubt face this mix up in priorities at judgment. Are we trading God's will for temporary pleasure?

*1 Timothy 4:7-8 But refuse profane and old wives' fables, and exercise thyself rather unto godliness. **For bodily exercise profiteth little:** but godliness is profitable unto all things, having promise of the life that now is, and of that which is to come.*

Yes even bodily exercise is mentioned in the Bible! It is second to exercising godliness however. What would it profit you to reach your ideal weight/shape but lose out on your spiritual inheritance? Let us deny our flesh and get to a healthy weight and honor God with our bodies, but let us not exchange obtaining health for salvation. We must not lose our focus on serving the Lord. We used to replace God with food and that got us overweight and further from Him. Now that we are on a different path, let us not put our desire to reach a certain weight/shape get in the way of our walk with God either.

*Matthew 16:24-28 Then said Jesus unto his disciples, If any man will come after me, let him deny himself, and take up his cross, and follow me. **For whosoever will save his life shall lose it: and whosoever will lose his life for my sake shall find it.** For what is a man profited, if he shall gain the whole world, and lose his own soul? or what shall a man give in exchange for his soul? For the Son of man shall come in the glory of his Father with his angels; and then he shall reward every man according to his works. Verily I say unto you, There be some standing here, which shall not taste of death, till they see the Son of man coming in his kingdom.*

If we find ourselves prioritizing our physical desires over the will of God we will be right back where we started in idolatry. In fact putting oneself on God's throne is the most common form of idolatry. Remember that if we are ever going to get healthy, God has to be involved. He is the one who heals and wounds.

Biblical Diet

Here are some of the healing foods mentioned in the Bible: apples, barley, cilantro, dates, figs, fish, garlic, grapes, honey, leeks, legumes, melons, milk, cheese, nuts, olives, onions, peppermint, wheat, yogurt, venison. It's no wonder they lived longer than we do now.

I leave you with this Scripture from Brother John.

2 John 1:2 Beloved, I wish above all things that thou mayest prosper and be in health, even as thy soul prospereth.

Minister Aaron Iacino

www.ingramcontent.com/pod-product-compliance
Lightning Source LLC
Chambersburg PA
CBHW071157280526
45787CB00002B/533